Psychiatric Interviewing and Assessment

Rob Poole
Consultant Psychiatrist, North East Wales Trust, Flintshire; Honorary Clinical
Lecturer, Department of Psychiatry, University of Liverpool, UK

Robert Higgo
Consultant Psychiatrist, Merseycare Trust, Liverpool, UK

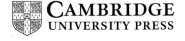

CAMBRIDGE
UNIVERSITY PRESS

CAMBRIDGE UNIVERSITY PRESS

Cambridge, New York, Melbourne, Madrid, Cape Town, Singapore, São Paulo
Cambridge University Press
The Edinburgh Building, Cambridge CB2 2RU, UK

Published in the United States of America by Cambridge University Press, New York

http://www.cambridge.org
Information on this title: www.cambridge.org/9780521671194

First published 2006
Reprinted 2006

Printed in the United Kingdom at the University Press, Cambridge

A catalogue record for this publication is available from the British Library

Library of Congress Cataloguing-in-Publication Data

Poole, Rob, 1956-
    Psychiatric interviewing and assessment / Rob Poole, Robert Higgo.
        p. ; cm.
    Includes bibliographical references and index.
    ISBN-13: 978-0-521-67119-4 (pbk.)
    ISBN-10: 0-521-67119-1 (pbk.)
    1. Interviewing in psychiatry. 2. Personality assessment. 3. Mental
status examination. I. Higgo, Robert, 1952- . II. Title.
[DNLM: 1. Interview, psychological – methods. 2. Mental disorders –
diagnosis. 3. Personality assessment. 4. Physician–patient relations.
    WM 141 P822p 2006]
    RC480.7.P62 2006
    616.89′075–dc22

                                                2005023717

ISBN-13 978-0-521-67119-4 paperback
ISBN-10 0-521-67119-1 paperback

Psychiatric Interviewing and Assessment

This book will help mental health professionals to develop the fundamental generic skills in interviewing and assessment, which form the foundation of psychiatric practice. It is about the process of reaching a diagnosis, and is a practical guide to help the reader make the transition from novice to competent clinician. It is based on real problems encountered in modern general adult psychiatric practice, and is set in a range of environments, in the clinic and in the community. The text is punctuated by a selection of case studies to illustrate the principles highlighted in the book.

This book will be essential reading for all members of the mental health team. Its practical grounding in everyday clinical experience will appeal to trainee psychiatrists and more experienced clinicians alike, as well as to nurses, social workers and psychologists.

Rob Poole is a community psychiatrist with an interest in the psychological, social and cultural aspects of mental illness. He has wide experience as a postgraduate educator having been a Royal College Clinical Tutor and Examiner, a University Postgraduate Tutor and Chairman of a regional psychiatric training committee.

Robert Higgo is the consultant psychiatrist for an Assertive Outreach Team in Liverpool, dealing with difficult to engage and complex client groups. He was a Royal College Tutor and Examiner, and Joint Programme Director for the Merseyside Rotational Training Scheme in Psychiatry.

This book is dedicated to **Dr Kevin White**.

There may be better psychiatric interviewers in the world, but we've never met one.

Contents

Acknowledgements

This book has a long history. We were originally brought together to work on a book for psychiatric trainees about clinical skills in 1996 by Dr Michael Göpfert. Although we have produced a book with a very different emphasis to his original idea, we are grateful to Michael for his encouragement in the early development of the project.

We have been greatly assisted by the comments of numerous trainees and colleagues, who have selflessly read various versions of the text (some of which, in retrospect, weren't very good). The book is a good deal easier to read as a consequence of their efforts, but they cannot be held responsible for our obstinate attachment to our opinions.

Dr Richard Barnes gave us invaluable assistance in preparing the chapter on cognitive state assessment. We are grateful to Dr Sue Ruben, who loaned us her cottage in Snowdonia, where the book was finally completed in the spring of 2005. She also painted the cover illustration.

This book is based upon our experience of treating a large number of patients, mainly in Liverpool. Most of what we know, we have learned from them. Their warmth and generosity in the face of some of the more difficult aspects of mental illness and psychiatric practice is a continuing source of inspiration.

Finally, and above all, this book could not have been completed without the support of our families, who have indulged us through long periods when publication appeared unlikely. The consequences for them have been far-reaching. The two families have converged to share uncomfortable but cheerful sailing holidays in Scotland, and the rather more mixed pleasures of supporting Manchester City Football Club.

Introduction

This book is intended to help mental health professionals to develop generic clinical skills in psychiatric interviewing and assessment. We have attempted to write a book that we would have found helpful at the beginning of our careers in clinical psychiatry, both in learning to do the job properly and in passing postgraduate examinations. The content is relevant to a range of mental health disciplines, including nursing, social work and psychology. We did consider writing the book from a multi-disciplinary point of view. However, from the outset we wanted to write a text that was readable and authentic. We have therefore addressed the book primarily to psychiatrists, as working as a psychiatrist is what we know best. We hope that this will not undermine the book's relevance to practitioners of other professions. Similarly, we have tended to use male pronouns generically, and there is a certain maleness in many of the vignettes. We hope that these accommodations to readability, and to our gender, do not give an impression of sexism.

This book is not about treatment, pharmacological or psychological. It is not about specialist assessments, such as the assessment of children and adults with learning disabilities, forensic assessment, neuropsychiatric evaluation or psycho-therapeutic assessment. It is about those fundamental generic skills that all psychiatrists need, and that form the foundation in developing more specialist skills.

The book assumes the level of knowledge of psychiatry necessary to qualify as a doctor or as a mental health nurse in the United Kingdom. We have tried to avoid the use of jargon as far as possible. The book has a general orientation towards community psychiatric practice, but it is theoretically eclectic and, as far as possible, evidence based. Where we have expressed opinions, or have taken a controversial point of view, we have tried to clearly indicate this. We have kept referencing to a minimum, as we believe it undermines readability. We have indicated a few other books that we think are particularly helpful.

This book is intended to be practical. It is a guide to clinical practice, and is built around situations that are readily recognisable from clinical experience. We have used clinical vignettes to illustrate principles throughout the book, and have taken great care to make these realistic. We have not used true stories. Our patients and colleagues may feel that they recognise themselves in the vignettes. If so, they are mistaken. If the stories seem familiar, it is because there are recurrent themes in clinical practice.

We have more than 45 years' clinical experience between us, much of this in 'hard end' inner city practice: in assertive outreach, amongst the homeless and in very deprived areas. This has taught us that the most important objective in psychiatry is to get alongside the patient. This does not mean doing whatever the patient wants. It means working towards an alliance whereby, together, the clinician and the patient can find a route to recovery. The task is embedded in everything that goes on between the professional and the patient; it cannot be neglected while some technical task is being completed. Furthermore, it can only be achieved if the clinician has an awareness of the importance of context and is able to understand the patient's point of view. It is true that this perspective demands some extra effort from the clinician early in his relationship with the patient. However, we have found that, overall, it takes less effort to do psychiatry well than to do it badly.

In order to write this book, we have had to reflect long and hard on our own clinical practice. We hope that this has not resulted in a text that is idiosyncratic and anecdotal, but that other experienced clinicians will recognise the processes and dilemmas that we have identified. The book has five overarching and interrelated themes, which are important in clinical practice. These are:

- Process: assessment is not just a series of questions to be asked but also a process between two people. Attention to the process optimises assessment and creates the foundations for a therapeutic alliance.
- Patient-centredness: understanding the patient as a person and understanding their subjective experience of their illness is an essential perspective in evaluating psychopathology, risk and so on. We explore the patient's experience of the interview through examination of the separate agendas of the professional and the patient. Resolving the tension between these agendas is a key task for the clinician.
- Context: we explore the impact of the patient's psychological and social context, the context of the interview and the professional's psychological and social background as important factors that can assist or interfere with assessment.
- Hypothesising: most textbooks suggest that assessment consists of information gathering and mental state examination followed by diagnosis or formulation. In fact, experienced clinicians operate by forming hypotheses and testing them throughout an assessment. This is an efficient, flexible and critical process. There are significant pitfalls for novices. If they fail to recognise that

they are likely to form impressions very early in interviews, then those impressions are not easily challenged. A conscious awareness of the hypothesising process makes for better assessments.

- Clinical scepticism: this is that essential critical and independent-minded quality that is shared by all good psychiatrists. It leads equally to a questioning of psychiatric orthodoxy and to an awareness that patients, their families and their friends all provide information that is affected by their subjective stand point.

The most useful psychiatric books are read as much for pleasure as for self-improvement. This book is intended to be a light read, but its objective is serious. We both feel that the process of writing the book has made us better, more reflective clinicians. If we help younger colleagues to become skilled clinicians without making as many mistakes as we did along the way, we shall be well pleased.

Part I

What am I trying to find out here?

There is a central and unavoidable problem at the heart of the work of all health professionals. The practice of medicine and allied professions is increasingly based on empirical science, generating interventions that are essentially technological and standardised. These technologies may be psychological, social or biological (or involve a combination of these modalities). However, the scientific-technological has to be applied in the context of patients' lives, an arena rich in complexity and ambiguity. At its simplest, no matter how effective a drug may be, it cannot work if the patient does not take it. The factors that make patients reluctant to accept advice may appear irrational to clinicians, but they are highly relevant to patients. No one can be expected to accept an intervention unless they are reasonably certain that the balance of the cost–benefit equation will lead to a positive change that is relevant to the quality of their life, as they understand it.

Much of this book is concerned with the development of the fundamental skills of forming and maintaining relationships with patients in order to deploy technologies without causing harm. This first section, however, is about a simultaneous, more technical task: the formation of a diagnostic understanding of the patient's problem, which is based primarily on history taking and mental state examination.

The objective of this section is to understand what one is looking for during assessment, and to explore some of the problems associated with the technical task.

1

Diagnosis

Is the medical model useful or valid?

'The medical model' is a puzzling concept. For many years, there has appeared to be a consensus that the medical model as applied to mental disorder is a bad thing, and for the most part only the most convinced biological psychiatrists have been prepared to defend it. However, it is far from clear as to what the term actually means. Sometimes it is used to mean the professional dominance of doctors within mental health care. On other occasions, it seems to mean institutional models of care. Most frequently, it is used to characterise a sterile, dehumanised, genetic-pharmacological stance that does exist within psychiatry, but which cannot be reasonably described as the mainstream. A telling definition of 'the medical model' was given to us by a clinical psychologist some years ago, which is that it is anything that doctors do. This is at least logical.

We are happy to defend *a* medical model, which remains in robust good health, despite decades of sustained criticism and attack from a wide variety of sources. We do recognise that it has limitations and contradictions, but it is the de facto model of mental health care across the world, and it is not going to go away. Furthermore, it has some strengths. No one, so far, has come up with an alternative that could plausibly be expected to improve our ability to help people with mental disorder.

Few people could work in health care without sometimes being embarrassed or angered by the actions of doctors, either because of individual shortcomings or because of institutional self-interest. However, no profession could defend itself on the basis of the activities of its worst practitioners. The underlying model of medicine is the application of objective science to help people in the context of their lives and environments; the scientific and human tasks are of equal importance. When medicine runs into trouble, it is usually because the two have become disconnected. Out of this medical model have sprung not just pharmacological and surgical treatments, but the whole of public health, including an understanding of the need for adequate hygiene, sanitation, nutrition and housing. The origins of psychotherapy and of social intervention to improve the health of the population lie within medicine. Where medicine has tried to impose crude technologies on patients, it has usually been based on poor (or even pseudo-) science, which is a betrayal of the fundamental task of the profession. The strength of medicine, and therefore the medical model, is its ability to understand problems at multiple levels simultaneously and to intervene in helpful ways that are informed, but not dominated, by scientific empiricism.

The limitations of diagnosis

Diagnosis lies at the heart of the medical model. It is a concept that unequivocally belongs to medicine and to the general medical approach to understanding human suffering. Embedded within the idea of diagnosis is an implicit assumption that symptoms, signs and natural history group together to form syndromes; that such syndromes can be understood at a physiological level; and that this can lead to the discovery of pathological processes and underlying causations. The movement of diagnosis from syndrome, to physiology, to pathology, to causation, has underpinned a substantial proportion of all progress in medicine. It has been particularly effective in understanding infectious diseases and finding treatments and preventive measures for them. Recently, it has underpinned the progress that has been made in responding to the global AIDS pandemic.

Sometimes, the same process has been effective in understanding mental disorders. In the nineteenth century, general paralysis of the insane (a type of neuro-syphilis) and some forms of complex partial epileptic seizures were regarded as part of an undifferentiated syndrome of 'insanity'. Now they are relatively well understood and can be treated with reference to underlying organic pathologies and physiological processes. In the last few years, this process has led to the identification and better understanding of Lewy body disease from amongst the dementias of old age. However, overall, diagnosis in psychiatry has yet to move significantly beyond the level of syndrome. Despite extensive research effort into the major syndromes (such as schizophrenia, bipolar affective disorder and depression), underlying physiologies, pathologies and causations remain elusive.

The lack of clear biological causations is probably not just the consequence of a lack of scientific knowledge. No matter how far we progress scientifically, some psychiatric problems are unlikely to prove to have a biological basis. When considered overall, psychiatric diagnosis is heterogeneous, embracing a wide diversity of disorders. This includes dementias (which definitely have a basis in coarse brain disease), psychoses (which probably have a fundamental basis in either brain dysfunction or subtle structural abnormalities), personality disorders (which are probably in large part developmental problems as a consequence of childhood adversity) and psychological reactions, which may arguably lie within the range of normal human experience. Clearly, the reductionist approach is unlikely to be useful in understanding or managing some of these problems.

A primary concern of patients is the development of effective, safe, tolerable and user-friendly treatments, and here recent progress has been relatively good. However, few treatments in psychiatry are specific to diagnosis. Generally speaking, our treatments are effective for particular symptoms. Antipsychotic drugs are useful in treating delusions and hallucinations, irrespective of diagnosis, and cognitive–behavioural therapy has been shown to be useful in treating virtually every major mental disorder, provided the symptoms make the patient either anxious or depressed. Some modern critics of psychiatric diagnosis (for example, Bentall, 1992) have argued that the whole nosology is illogical, unscientific and should be abandoned. It is argued that we should focus on specific problems rather than diagnoses. Whilst this stance has an iconoclastic appeal, it ignores the secure knowledge that we do possess, which has important practical and scientific implications. We do have an excellent understanding of the ways in which symptoms group together, the courses that such syndromes generally follow, some of the ways in which these disorders develop and the factors that tend to relieve or exacerbate them.

Until the 1970s it was more difficult to defend psychiatric diagnosis, as, frankly, the nosology was a mess. A series of well-known international studies (for example, Cooper *et al.*, 1972) showed that, whilst the prevalence of the major psychoses was remarkably similar in different countries, psychiatrists had entirely different definitions for the same disorders, and consequently there was not a common international psychiatric language. At this stage, psychiatric diagnosis could be criticised for lacking even semantic validity.

There were also idiosyncratic diagnostic systems in various countries, and diagnostic concepts came under critical scrutiny. One of the repetitive errors of psychiatry has been to base diagnosis on supposed, but unproven, causations. A key example was the distinction in the UK between 'endogenous' and 'reactive' depression. Endogenous depression was said to arise, without psychological or social antecedents, from within the person (probably owing to a genetic factor) and was said to be severe and characterised by biological symptoms. Reactive depression was less severe and closely related to the person's circumstances. Vulnerability was believed to be related to social stress and personality. Unfortunately, this neat distinction fell apart when studied closely (for example, Kendell, 1976). The presence of biological symptoms turned out to be a reflection of the severity of depression, and stressors were shown to be equally important at either end of the severity spectrum. Not only did symptoms fail to cluster into two neat groups, it was also more difficult than expected even to demonstrate that anxiety and depression were two separate syndromes.

The development of the International Classification of Diseases, Tenth Edition (WHO, 1992) (itself influenced by the development of successive Diagnostic and Statistical Manuals in the USA) has at least elevated psychiatric diagnosis to the level where categories have some basis in demonstrable syndromes. This classification (universally known as ICD-10) is a multi-axial diagnostic system with operational criteria for various diagnostic categories. It has been shown to have at least face validity and clinical utility. We now share an international scientific language that can be readily understood by reference to an accessible and understandable glossary. Indeed, the ICD-10 glossary is essential reading. It is well written, clear and includes explanations of the nature of the categories. There are still unresolved controversies, and even within a more evidence-based nosology, we retain diagnoses that take putative causation, rather than symptom clusters, as their starting point (e.g. post-traumatic stress disorder). Given the state of development of psychiatry as a science, ICD-10 can only be regarded as provisional, and it will be revised and replaced in due course. It is useful as long as one recognises the limitations to its application.

ICD-10 is like a map. It provides a model for understanding the relationship between different disorders. It tells patients and clinicians where an individual's mental health problem lies within the whole psychiatric terrain. It tells you little or nothing about the person and their life; like a map, it does not necessarily tell you much beyond generalities.

Beyond diagnosis

Psychiatry has recognised the inadequacies of using diagnosis in isolation for a very long time. British psychiatry, largely under the influence of Sir Aubrey Lewis, traditionally emphasised the need to develop a 'formulation' of each case. This was a detailed understanding of the contextual factors, biological, psychological and social, which had predisposed, precipitated and perpetuated a patient's disorder. It was recognised that diagnosis was of limited usefulness at the level of helping people. The importance of the formulation was that it gave a far more detailed understanding, and could guide treatment. The term fell from use quite suddenly when British psychiatrists were asked what should be included in a formulation, and there was no general agreement. As a consequence, the term was dropped from the British postgraduate examinations, and was replaced by the term 'assessment'. This has an identical function to formulation, and no doubt if a contemporary study was conducted, there would still be no general agreement.

In our opinion, this reflects the difficulty in operationalising that which is obvious. The diversity of factors that may be important at a human level is such that it is impossible to make a single statement as to what should be included and, more importantly, what should be left out. Assessment has to include the patient's concerns and those pressures, weaknesses and strengths operating in their lives, because these are the factors that are most important in finding a path to recovery. Ways of understanding mental disorder that avoid meaning at a human level are essentially sterile and are of very limited helpfulness. It seems self-evident that disorders that affect feelings, thinking and behaviour have an important dimension of meaningfulness; not obscure or unconscious meaning, but a more accessible emotional and practical meaning. Whilst it may be useful at times to think of mental disorders as arising within the brain or the mind, the location of the problem is actually in peoples' lives.

ICD-10 attempts to deal with this difficulty by having five axes (see Box 1.1). This does allow a more comprehensive, operationally defined, description of a problem, and does clearly allow for the fact that personality disorder is a risk factor for mental illness, not a mutually exclusive diagnosis. However, the system is only useful administratively. In the clinical situation, a list of categorically organised problems, stripped of all context and meaning, is of little help.

An alternative approach to both formulation and multi-axial classification is the use of problem lists. This has been developed, for the most part, by clinicians with an interest in cognitive–behavioural therapy (CBT), and it closely follows the intellectual traditions of that approach. It is not suggested that problem lists should replace diagnosis. The problem list is a tool, sitting alongside diagnosis and providing a way of breaking complex difficulties down into a series of discrete identifiable problems, each of which can be tackled with reference to an action plan. A problem list might look something like Box 1.2.

Problem lists have an attractive commonsense quality, and lend themselves to clear monitoring of progress. Most clinicians use some form of problem list to organise interventions, even if the list is not formalised in this way. There are potential pitfalls to the approach. Breaking problems down can lead to a loss of long-term and thematic perspectives, in other words breaking things down too

---

BOX 1.1 ICD-10 axes

Axis I: Mental disorder (e.g. syndromic mental illness)

Axis II: Developmental disorder (e.g. personality disorder)

Axis III: Intellectual impairment (e.g. learning disability)

Axis IV: Physical disorder

Axis V: Psychosocial problems

BOX 1.2 A problem list

Mrs. A, a 53-year-old woman with late-onset paranoid schizophrenia.

Problem 1. Auditory, tactile and olfactory hallucinations and paranoid delusions regarding neighbours.

Action 1.   Consultant psychiatrist to arrange treatment with antipsychotic medication.

Problem 2. Reluctant to take medication owing to limited insight into the nature of the problem.

Action 2.   Community mental health nurse to carry out insight directed/concordance therapy.

Problem 3. Conflict with neighbours owing to arguments based on paranoid delusions.

Action 3.   Social worker to organise rehousing for patient and her husband.

Problem 4. Psychosis worsened by worries over debts.

Action 4.   Social worker to organise referral to welfare rights worker to maximise state benefits and to assist with debt management.

Problem 5. Conflict with daughters, who have been unable to comprehend their mother's behaviour.

Action 5.   Community mental health nurse to conduct psychoeducational sessions with the family.

---

much can drain the meaningful connections between individual problems. As far as possible, problem lists need to be developed with the patient, not imposed on them, as they can turn into a paternalistic and disempowering programme. Some clinicians (including ourselves) feel that they overlook the importance of more subtle, but important, factors arising out of relationships with individual clinicians that can contribute to (or impede) recovery.

There are many other approaches to the task of producing a concise, coherent account of the important features of a patient's disorder in the context of their life. Like many experienced clinicians, our preference is a narrative, a story that draws all the threads together so that we, and the patient, can understand what has happened to them, set in a chronological framework. This preference may simply reflect our personalities, but we believe that it has real advantages. We find that a narrative is easier to remember, and easier to convey verbally to other professionals. However, the important thing is to find an approach to formulation that works for oneself and one's patients.

Diagnostic uncertainty

At the end of an assessment interview, it is conventional for the psychiatrist to write out a differential diagnosis. This is a list of the main diagnostic possibilities, listed in order of decreasing likelihood. It may include both diagnostic alternatives and additional diagnoses. In the UK, differential diagnosis is pragmatic. It should include only what is plausible, not every conceivable possibility, no matter how unlikely. In some countries, exhaustive thoroughness is highly valued, but the whole British medical tradition rejects this as unfocused and unhelpful.

The differential diagnostic process is reflective of the fact that even the most thorough assessment is unlikely to generate diagnostic certainty. Diagnostic uncertainty can persist for years, though usually it can be resolved reasonably promptly. However, an excessive impatience to make a firm diagnosis leads, over time, to patients accumulating multiple diagnostic labels, which is confusing for everyone. Diagnostic uncertainty has to be managed, as it cannot be eliminated.

For obvious reasons, the commonest, and most easily resolved, cause of uncertainty is lack of information, which itself plays against the backdrop of the diagnostic hierarchy in psychiatry (see Box 1.3). The diagnostic hierarchy has to be considered, no matter what system of diagnosis and formulation is used. The principle is that conditions higher up the hierarchy can cause symptoms of conditions lower down the hierarchy. The most important point is that all psychiatric disorders, no matter how typically they may present, can be caused by underlying physical disease. This means that there is *always* a degree of uncertainty, as physical disease is not always detectable, even with the use of the full range of physical investigations.

In other respects, the hierarchy is not 100% reliable. One could argue at length as to whether personality disorder should appear in the hierarchy at all. It is included mainly because quite convincing presentations of personality disorder can turn out to be due to other disorders. For example, apparent antisocial personality can arise in the context of chronic low-grade hypomania. Obviously, this diagnostic error would be likely to occur in the absence of comprehensive information, but we all work in an imperfect world, where significant

---

BOX 1.3 The diagnostic hierarchy in psychiatry

1. Coarse physical brain disorder
2. Psychotic disorder (schizophrenia, bipolar affective disorder, persistent delusional disorder, depression with delusions)
3. Personality disorder
4. Depression without delusions
5. Anxiety states

decisions must sometimes be made without as much information as one would like.

Hypotheses and cumulative certainty

A theme of this book, and indeed of all mental health practice, is hypothesising. Diagnoses, and much else, exist as clinical hypotheses, which must be continuously tested. In particular, when something happens, or information comes to light, which does not fit with usual patterns, clinical hypotheses have to be reconsidered. Related to this is the concept of cumulative certainty, the process by which a particular diagnosis or formulation becomes increasingly (but not necessarily absolutely) certain. This is codified in some particularly tricky diagnostic areas. Long before operationalised diagnostic criteria emerged, psychiatrists had difficulty in clearly distinguishing schizophrenia from other psychoses and severe affective disorders. Kurt Schneider developed the concept of 'first rank symptoms' (Schneider, 1959), which is to say a group of symptoms that are particularly characteristic of schizophrenia (see Box 1.4). Whilst all of them can arise in other disorders, the more that are present, the more likely it is that the patient is suffering from schizophrenia. This system has been evaluated against more modern approaches, and whilst contemporary research criteria are more reliable, it stands up remarkably well (Kendell *et al.*, 1979). First rank symptoms continue to have a clinical usefulness.

Similarly, there was long-standing controversy as to where the boundary between normal drinking and alcoholism lay, together with difficulties in defining severity of alcohol dependency problems (see Box 1.5). Edwards and Gross devised the alcohol dependency syndrome (Edwards and Gross, 1976) with explicit reference to Schneider's first rank symptoms. Rejecting a clear boundary between normal and problem drinking, they identified seven key features. The more the patient displays, the more severe the problem. After thirty years, this remains a helpful clinical tool.

BOX 1.4 Schneider's first rank symptoms of schizophrenia

- Delusional perception
- Third person auditory hallucinations, including running commentary
- Somatic hallucinations
- Disorders of the possession of thought (hearing one's thoughts spoken out loud, thought insertion, thought withdrawal, thought broadcasting)
- Passivity experiences (thoughts, actions and emotions experienced as literally under the control of an external agency)

> **BOX 1.5 Alcohol dependency syndrome**
> - Salience/primacy of alcohol consumption
> - Craving/compulsion to take alcohol
> - Tolerance of the effects of intoxication (or loss of tolerance at a late stage)
> - Repeated episodes of withdrawal symptoms
> - Relief drinking to control withdrawal symptoms ('eye-openers')
> - Narrowing of drinking repertoire
> - Repeated reinstatement of drinking after abstinence

Stigma

In psychiatry, diagnosis has a profound effect upon the patient. Many patients feel that the social stigma attached to their diagnosis is more problematic than the symptoms of the illness itself. 'I have diabetes' or 'I have asthma' are statements that have implications for an individual's lifestyle and even their life expectancy. Such diagnoses can cause significant problems, for example, in obtaining life insurance at a reasonable premium. However, these statements, made in a social setting, have only a limited impact on the sufferer's relationship with the rest of the world. The disclosure 'I have manic-depression', on the other hand, is likely to cause an irrevocable shift in a social relationship, and often the shift is in an unwelcome direction. Even if the diagnosis is later withdrawn because it has turned out to be wrong, the patient's previous relationship with the rest of the world is not restored. 'At first they said I had thyrotoxicosis, but apparently I haven't after all' has an entirely different impact to 'At first they said I had schizophrenia, but apparently I haven't after all'. These problems of social stigma cannot be dismissed or ignored. Patients justifiably complain that a psychiatric diagnosis is a burdensome label, which leads to loss of autonomy and to social marginalisation.

As a consequence of this, some clinicians are reluctant to make the most socially stigmatising diagnoses at all. Many more are reluctant to share such diagnoses with their patients and their families. This solves no problems, and indeed can amount to a betrayal of the fundamental duty of truthfulness. Patients and families frequently complain of a lack of diagnosis. Once reasonable care has been made to make a full assessment (which can take some time), a clearly explained diagnostic formulation, including an explanation of such ambiguities and uncertainties as exist, is essential. It allows people to understand what has happened to them, to access as much information as they need and to secure assistance from non-health care agencies such as the voluntary sector and self-help groups. All of these can be crucial in helping people to regain control of their lives.

Over many decades euphemisms have been introduced to try and reduce stigma. Attempts to replace 'mental handicap' with 'learning disability' and 'mental illness' with 'mental distress' are just two recent examples. If patients prefer these terms, we should respect their choice, but objectively speaking, there is little evidence that they have achieved much in reducing stigma. Stigma rests not in words, but in social attitudes, themselves based on ignorance and fear. In the UK, politicians and the media have tended to exacerbate stigma by an expedient recourse to crude and inappropriate stereotypes. As clinicians we have three duties with respect to the stigma attached to the diagnoses we make: to recognise that diagnosis tangibly affects our patients' lives; to eliminate stigmatising attitudes from our own practice; and to be part of a wide alliance to combat stigma in the general public. At the most basic level we should recognise that our patients are not, for example, schizophrenics, but people suffering from schizophrenia.

Main points in this chapter

1. Diagnosis has a role in understanding mental disorder, but it has problems and limitations.
2. Diagnosis is insufficient on its own to allow us to understand patients' problems.
3. No person can be defined or fully described by a diagnosis.
4. The problems with psychiatric diagnosis are also evident in other areas of medicine, though they may be less immediately obvious elsewhere.

History

What is the point of history taking?

The whole of the practice of psychiatry rests upon access to a reliable and comprehensive history. No one can expect to safely treat any patient without a good understanding of how they have come to develop this problem at this time. Without knowledge of their lifestyle, concerns, strengths and weaknesses, attempts at intervention are likely to be clumsy and inappropriate. Obtaining a full history is by far and away the single most important task in psychiatric assessment. It is of considerably greater value than more technically complex tasks such as mental state examination, cognitive assessment or physical investigations, though each of these are important in their own right. Mental state examination, for example, is essentially a snap shot located in a moment in time. Consequently, if too much reliance is placed upon it in making a diagnosis, it can be misleading. Mental state examination needs the context provided by history to be meaningful.

All mental health professionals make errors from time to time. In our experience, errors most often occur because the history is inadequate. One might suppose that this usually happens when patients first come into contact with mental health services, as decisions often have to be made before comprehensive information is available. In fact, at this stage, most professionals are aware of the ambiguities caused by lack of information, and tend to be appropriately cautious as a consequence. Problems more frequently arise when patients have been in contact with services for a while. Continuing history taking is sometimes neglected because the person is 'well known'. Sometimes, parts of the patient's history have not been properly understood or have been forgotten; and sometimes, something new and important has happened, but the professionals miss it because no one thinks it necessary to ask. It is self-evident that no one can ever know everything about another person. The objective, therefore, is to collate an adequate history, but to bear in mind that the task is never really complete.

History taking is not a passive process of information collection. It is an active and continuing process, which involves understanding and organising information. This chapter is not about the process of obtaining a history, which is dealt with elsewhere in this book. Here, we are concerned with the information that needs to be collected and how it should be organised. Clearly, the emphasis and detail needed varies in different situations, but the main components of an adequate history are, for the most part, invariable.

The proforma has become an increasingly prominent part of clinical practice in recent years. A proforma can provide a useful aide memoire for history taking, though forms are a very awkward method of keeping records. Spaces tend to be too small or too big, and there is a perverse incentive to cover parts of history with a generalisation, rather than detail. It can be very difficult to retrieve information from standardised forms. Proformas can dictate the way that an interview is conducted, leading the interviewer to interrogate the patient and impose excessive control over the direction of the discussion. Needless to say, we do not like assessment proforma much, as we feel that they cause more problems than they solve. Leaving aside these practical considerations, they remind us of the pre-war admission sheets which could be found in the case notes of long-stay patients in large mental hospitals. These were elderly people who lived barren, institutional lives for decades, having been first admitted as young people. The admission sheets, on heavy foolscap paper with copperplate handwriting and a faded photograph, seemed to signify the reduction of the patient's life to an administrative procedure.

Despite these unpleasant resonances and limitations in practice, assessment forms are part of modern health-care culture. If proformas must be used, it is best to interview the patient in the normal way, and to fill in the forms retrospectively.

General considerations

Box 2.1 sets out the basic structure of a psychiatric history. A reasonably straightforward initial assessment might generate a history following this general outline and with information under each of the headings. Various authorities have suggested that histories should be set out in different orders, but the headings rarely differ. This is the structure that we have found most useful in general adult psychiatric practice. It lends itself to later amendment and expansion. We sometimes follow this structure in an interview, but not always. As we discuss later, this is a structure for organising histories, not interviews. In particular, history taking and mental state examination are not, in the real world, fully separate tasks, but are usually recorded separately.

The structure covers all aspects of the patient's life, and forms a kind of abbreviated biography. Very few people think about themselves and their lives in

---

> **BOX 2.1 The basic structure of a psychiatric history**
> - Reason for referral
> - History of presenting problem
> - Psychiatric history
> - Family history
> - Childhood history
> - Educational history
> - Occupational history
> - Sexual and reproductive history
> - Medical history
> - Social history and daily routines
> - Substance misuse history
> - Forensic history
> - Pre-morbid personality

---

this structured biographical way. Consequently, constructing a chronology is an essential task when organising the information one is given. Gaps in chronology, in other words periods when it is not clear what was happening in the person's life, are important. They demand further inquiry. Histories should either be organised around the patient's age at the time, or the date, whichever the patient finds easier. Without this, gaps will go unnoticed. Combinations of date and age are confusing, and are to be avoided if possible.

There is a general principle that it is far more illuminating to ask people about the tangible than about the abstract. For example, asking the patient why his marriage broke up invites a general, and uninformative, answer, for example, 'I wasn't very happy in the marriage and we drifted apart', whereas asking what happened, about the events that provoked the divorce, focuses on the particular, and is more likely to reveal reasons. Although one is concerned with the patient's feelings, what actually has happened in their life is the basis of a good history.

Reason for referral

In psychiatry, very few things happen suddenly. Most people have been struggling with their problem for months, or even years, before they finally come for help. How they came to be sitting in front of you is relevant both to the here and now of the interview, and in understanding the overall situation. Did they come of their own volition, or did they come under duress? Why have they come now, rather than last week or a month ago? Why did the referrer think the patient needed assessment? What events provoked the request for assessment? The answers to these questions reveal the concerns of the patient and the concerns of those around them. It is especially important to elicit and record this information when people are assessed out of hours or in emergency situations, not least because it can be impossible to retrospectively find out what has gone on.

History of the presenting problem

The point here is to understand what is worrying the patient, and to understand how the problem has developed. What symptoms and behaviours are most concerning the patient and those around them? When did they start? Did any events or stresses seem to provoke or exacerbate the problem? What effect is the problem having on the patient's daily functioning? Can they cope with their job? Are they looking after their children properly? Are there changes in their motivation to do things that they enjoy or that they feel are important? What have their family and friends done in response to the problem?

Are they sleeping well? If not, they may be unable to drop off to sleep, or they may wake early. Sleep may be light with recurrent waking. Their sleep pattern may have reversed, with napping by day and wakefulness at night. Sleep is hard to assess, as broken sleep is often experienced as continuous wakefulness, which can lead people to believe that they are not sleeping at all. It is important to find out when they go to bed and when they rise. What do they do when they cannot sleep? On the one hand, getting up for a cigarette and a cup of tea worsens sleeplessness; on the other hand, people who lie awake all night in darkness and silence are probably sleeping more than they realise.

Has their eating pattern changed? Are there corresponding changes in their weight? A lot of people do not weigh themselves regularly, but nearly everyone notices when clothes become tighter or looser.

Is their concentration affected? The question is not always meaningful to people who do not have to absorb a lot of information every day. However, poor concentration is often experienced as forgetfulness. It takes a fair degree of concentration to follow the plot line of the average episode of a television soap opera. Questions about changes in concentration should not be an abstract inquiry, but need to relate to those intellectual tasks that arise regularly in people's lives.

Some would include a general question regarding mood and suicidal thoughts here, if they have not arisen as part of the description of the main problem. In the sequence of the interview they are often dealt with next. We discuss them under mental state examination, as that is where they logically belong. However, what does belong here is any history of self-harming behaviour, the circumstances under which it occurred, what the patient had expected to occur as a consequence and what did actually occur as a consequence. Assessment of suicidality is dealt with in Chapter 16.

Is there anything that the patient has found to help how they feel? Has their family doctor (GP), or anyone else, tried to treat them? Did it make any difference? If medication was prescribed, did they take it?

Psychiatric history

This includes both whether the patient has ever seen a mental health professional before, and whether they have experienced symptoms (whether similar to the current symptoms or not) prior to the current episode. Previous treatments and their outcome (including whether the patient experienced them as helpful) are obviously relevant. It is especially important to ask about previous psychiatric admissions, the length of the stay and whether the patient was subject to legal compulsion. Dates, locations and names of professionals are important in obtaining old records.

Family history

Though it is relevant to ask if other family members have suffered from mental health problems, family history is much more than this. It is important to ascertain the structure of the patient's family of origin. This includes parents' current ages, occupation, and the quality of the patient's relationship with each of them. Where parents have separated or one or both parents have died, the parent's and the patient's ages at the time are important reference points for the rest of the history. Ages of siblings, current relationship and a brief outline of their circumstances are also important. Where family structures are complex, it can be helpful to draw a schematic family tree.

We have found that many people confuse step-siblings (i.e. non-biological relationships with the offspring of step-parents) with half-siblings (i.e. those who share one parent). Equally, there is confusion between step-parent (the partner of a biological parent) with foster parents (adults who care for children on a temporary basis, often, but not always, as a job). Both of these are confused with adoptive parents (adults who take on full legal responsibility for children but are not biologically related to them). Each of these relationships has different implications, and drawing a clear distinction between them can be important.

Childhood history

Whilst some people can spontaneously give detailed accounts of their childhood, this is rarely possible for people who have experienced disrupted and disturbing childhoods. Whilst this is not surprising, given that it can be difficult to make sense of an unhappy childhood as you live through it, these are actually the childhood histories that are most important to understand. It is conventional to ask about developmental milestones (ages of first walking, talking, reading etc.), but in our experience, hardly anyone knows the answer unless there has been marked delay. Similarly, we were taught to ask about 'childhood neurotic traits', such as thumb-sucking and nail biting, but no one has ever explained to us what these behaviours mean. These problems are widespread in the population and they are of little significance. It is, however, worth asking about bed-wetting, as this can persist to adulthood, with a major impact on self-esteem.

What is more important is early losses and separations, any history of violence in the home and the patient's recollection of periods of persistent childhood unhappiness. The general rule about concentrating on the specific is particularly true here. Statements that a childhood has been unhappy tend to mean that the patient felt different to other children. They reflect a comparison. You need to know about events and family behaviours. This may involve direct questions about specific types of difficulties. Questions around these issues will frequently uncover histories of emotional or physical abuse (sexual abuse is usually best dealt with as part of sexual history, though people increasingly spontaneously disclose it, often as a consequence of being upset by coverage of the issue in the media).

Educational history

Educational histories are best divided into the main educational phases, that is primary school, secondary school and higher education. The types of school attended are relevant, together with changes of school and reasons for them. Peer relationships at school, especially any history of bullying or being bullied, disciplinary problems, truancy and school refusal should all be subject to inquiry if they are not volunteered. Academic attainment, including grades of any qualifications, should be ascertained. Where there is evidence of educational problems, it is worth directly asking about special schooling and referrals to child psychiatrists or educational psychologists. Under these circumstances, it is important to ask about literacy. Problems with reading and writing are far more widespread than is generally acknowledged, and can occur in otherwise intelligent people. Illiteracy tends to be accompanied by shame. 'Have you ever had problems with reading and writing?' captures the full range of difficulties, past and present. 'Can you read and write?' has an entirely different connotation, as illiteracy is rarely absolute, and invites a misleading and defensive reaction.

Occupational history

For most people, occupation (like relationships and reproduction) is one of the main reference points by which they structure an understanding of their life. A significant proportion of people with severe mental disorders have little or no experience of work, which is a major contributing factor in their social marginalisation. Where patients have an occupational history, the detail needed depends on how frequently job changes have occurred. If a middle-aged man has worked as a building labourer, then the nature of the work is usually casual and temporary, and he is unlikely to remember details of each job. Asking whether he has been sacked from jobs is more relevant. Less frequent changes, and promotions, can be important in more settled employment histories. Recurrent disputes with employers or workmates, or episodes of being bullied, are important. They may not be volunteered unless you ask whether the patient enjoyed the job, and if not, why not.

Sexual and reproductive history

The first issue in any sexual history is sexual orientation. Usually this becomes obvious from discussion early in interviews, but not always. A significant proportion of insecure heterosexual men can become surprisingly upset if one asks them if they are gay. They take the question as an affront to their masculinity, as they hope that their heterosexuality is self-evident. The question has to be put tactfully, by asking the patient to confirm their heterosexuality rather than to deny homosexuality. The trouble with avoiding the question is that it becomes more difficult to ask later on. Asking the question can become more offensive to the homophobe after you've had a chance to get to know them, as it becomes a deeper assault on their sexual identity.

Apart from this, one is trying to understand the person's history of serious (and therefore usually sexual) relationships; the quality of their current relationship, and what has gone wrong in past relationships. This may or may not lead to exploration of actual sexual problems. Age of puberty and of first sexual contact is generally relevant. Age of menopause and whether relationships are still sexually active is relevant in older people.

It is usually appropriate to ask a general question as to whether the person has had unwanted sexual experiences. Asked in this way, histories of childhood sexual abuse and rape may be volunteered. It is important not to press people into early disclosure of bad sexual experiences, as making such a disclosure to a stranger can be traumatising and unhelpful. The point is to indicate that the issue is available for discussion. Many people make disclosures in later interviews after initial denials, having had a chance to think about it and prepare themselves.

The modern concern with sexual abuse has tended to reduce focus on the importance of reproductive histories. Clearly, one wants, in all cases, to know about patients' children, their current circumstances and so on. Occasionally, this can be important in identifying child protection concerns. However, lost pregnancies, whether through miscarriage or medical termination, are important events. They are often overlooked unless one asks women how many times they have been pregnant before asking how many children they have.

Medical history

Current health problems and past illness, including hospital admissions and operations, should be recorded in detail. Patients should be asked what medication they are taking; drug names and dosages should be recorded, if possible. This is different from asking what they are being prescribed. Lists of medication in referral letters only tell you what the referrer thinks the patient is taking. The entire general population is not very compliant with intended drug regimes, and any doctor who thinks that their patients usually follow their instructions with regard to drug treatments is not asking patients about their use of medication in the right way. People should be asked about allergies; although this will elicit information about a host of non-allergic adverse responses to all kinds of agents, it is the only way to ensure that one knows about potentially life-threatening reactions.

Social history and daily routines

Social history is about the person's daily life at present. What type of housing do they have? Who owns the accommodation? Who is in the household? This may not be immediately obvious. Do they have friends and a social life? Have they given up social activities or contact with friends lately? Are there financial problems? If so, how did debts arise? What are their interests or hobbies? Some people deny any hobbies or interests, in which case it can be illuminating to ask what newspaper they read (if any), what television programmes they like and their taste in books or music.

Daily routines reveal a lot about a person's functioning. Simple questions, 'How do you spend your time each day?' and 'How did you spend your time before you became ill?' will usually elicit the information. Where a patient cannot, for whatever reason, answer these questions, it can be helpful to get them to describe a 24-hour period hour by hour, usually through describing the previous day.

Substance misuse

Substance misuse is extremely common amongst people with mental health problems. Whilst some types of substance misuse, especially alcohol misuse, can be the primary cause of mental ill health, more commonly it is a dysfunctional strategy to deal with feeling bad, which unfortunately tends to exacerbate the problem. The media, policy makers and providers of mental health services have been preoccupied with the problem of drug misuse for years. Whilst the problems caused by drugs are serious, this preoccupation has tended to obscure the range of substances that are misused. Furthermore, a far larger proportion of the population misuse alcohol than misuse drugs, and legal but heavy alcohol use can have considerably worse effects on a person's mental health than illegal but occasional use of drugs.

Quite apart from tobacco, alcohol and recreational drug use, one should bear in mind a number of other possibilities. The misuse of prescription drugs (especially benzodiazepines) is common. Over the counter medicines are also misused. Caffeine tablets are remarkably potent, as are proprietary cough medicines. Solvent misuse still occurs, primarily, but not exclusively, in teenagers. The cult of female thinness is matched by a corresponding male preoccupation with muscle bulk. The use of anabolic steroids and other, less reliable, anabolic agents is commonplace in gym culture. Herbal remedies are generally perceived as 'natural' and therefore safe, but they can be highly potent and quite toxic in large doses. Specific communities use substances that are unfamiliar to the rest of the population. For example, ghat (or khat) is a shrub that grows in East Africa. The leaves are chewed by men in the Somali and Yemeni communities. It has much the same effect as amphetamine, and causes similar problems with heavy use. It is currently legal in the UK. There are many other examples of less well known abusable substances.

Clearly, it is neither practical nor desirable to ask every patient about every potentially abusable substance. Questions about less common types of substance misuse are triggered by clues, and largely rest upon the professional's knowledge of the patterns of substance misuse. A young man who reports going to the gym regularly should be asked about steroids, but there is little point in asking the same question to an elderly woman. This is not the same as allowing one's assumptions to replace appropriate questions. Not all heavy drinkers look like stereotypical alcoholics, and there are people with alcohol problems even amongst devout religious communities that prohibit alcohol use completely.

Practically speaking, obtaining a substance misuse history rests on a combination of routine questions and pursuing clues from history and mental state examination. For example, it is quite difficult to accidentally burn the end of your nose, unless you use crack cocaine (commonly turned to vapour using a flame; the crack and the flame tend to be held in the direct vicinity of the nose). A burn to the tip of the nose invites a direct question. Similarly, it is reasonable to assume that anyone who attends an appointment smelling of alcohol has a drink problem, no matter how vehemently this is denied. Drinking before a serious meeting breaks a social taboo, and thus reflects the salience of drinking. The fact that this may be an attempt to control the anxiety generated by the meeting does not alter the fact that this is problem drinking. A smell of alcohol, lingering from the night before, reflects very heavy consumption, and one can safely assume that someone who claims they had 'a couple of glasses of wine' is either fooling themselves or has a very loose definition of 'a couple'. If someone close to you has suggested that you drink too much, you almost certainly have a problem. A conviction for drunk driving invariably indicates an alcohol problem.

In routine histories, one should ask how much tobacco the patient uses, and this is, of course, straightforward. Alcohol is more difficult. The probe 'Do you drink alcohol?' is less useful than 'How much do you drink?' or 'how much alcohol do you take?' This follows the general principle that, when asking about common behaviours which are socially embarrassing or seen as shameful, it is usually best to avoid structuring questions in such a way that there is an element of confession in the answer. Framing the question around the assumption that the person does drink is unlikely to offend the non-drinker and makes it easier for the drinker to open up. Similarly, the probe 'How much cannabis do you use?' is useful with people under forty. Cannabis use is common and attracts relatively little social opprobrium. Cannabis can cause quite severe problems in its own right, but is likely to be perceived as innocuous.

Whilst the majority of people who use cannabis do not use other drugs, nearly all serious drug users use cannabis. People who have never used cannabis are highly unlikely to have ever used other illegal drugs. Confirmation of cannabis use therefore opens up more detailed questioning about other drugs. However, in the case of drug use, the more direct approach can be effective. The question 'Have you ever used drugs?' does usually seem to generate a truthful answer, though it can shock people who are socially conservative. Contrary to their reputation,

---

BOX 2.2 A menu of specific questions in drug and alcohol histories

Alcohol

- At what age did you start drinking?
- Exactly how much did you drink yesterday, and at what times?
- Which brand, and what strength, of beer/cider do you drink?
- Do you drink wine as well? Do you ever drink spirits?
- Exactly what did you drink on your worst day this month?
- How much do you spend on alcohol? Where does the money come from?
- Have you ever been convicted of drunk-driving?
- Do other people think your drinking is a problem? Do you agree?
- Has your tolerance increased? Do you shake or retch in the mornings?
- Have you ever tried to give up drinking? What made you try?
- Have you had accidents when drunk or suffered from memory blackouts?
- Have you ever had a fit or hallucinations when you stopped drinking?
- What about drugs?

Drugs

- At what age did you start using drugs?
- What drugs have you ever used, and what do you use now?
- How do you pay for it? Do you owe money to a drug supplier?
- Have you ever injected drugs?
- Have you ever had a bad drug experience? Or had withdrawal symptoms?
- Do you think drugs cause you any problems?
- Which of the following do you use?
  Heroin, methadone, pharmaceutical opiates, benzodiazepines, cocaine, crack-cocaine, amphetamine, ketamine, LSD, magic mushrooms, ecstasy (and its analogues), cannabis, exotic drugs (e.g. khat).
- What about alcohol?

---

the vast majority of drug users are disarmingly frank about their habits. People who drink too much, on the other hand, have a strong tendency to minimise their consumption. This is related to a key feature of alcohol misuse, denial; drinkers tend to mislead themselves.

We have dwelt on substance misuse histories at some length, both because they are important and also because they present real difficulties. Box 2.2 sets out a menu of questions, not to be used as a rigid schema but to illustrate some useful lines of inquiry. No history taking technique is completely reliable and one has to maintain a relatively high level of suspicion that there may be an undisclosed substance misuse problem, no matter how well one knows the patient.

Forensic history

This refers to the patient's history of criminality. People with mental health problems are no more likely to offend than the general public, though career criminals who become mentally ill often become less adept at their art and are caught more frequently as a consequence. However, a substantial proportion of the population have at least one conviction. Men are more frequently convicted than women, and much more frequently imprisoned.

The probe 'Have you ever been in trouble with the law?' is fairly neutral, and seems not to offend the law-abiding. Not all prosecutions result in a conviction, and asking only about the patient's criminal record may miss important patterns of offending. Ideally, one should record the date of each prosecution, the exact offence (if the patient can remember), the circumstances leading to the prosecution and any penalty imposed. Some people have enormous criminal records for petty offending, in which case it may be more relevant to ask about convictions outside of their usual pattern, for example, whether a habitual shoplifter has any convictions for aggression. People who have convictions should be asked about similar behaviour that has not come to the attention of the criminal justice system, in other words, how often they have got away with it.

Pre-morbid personality

Medical students are taught to ask patients what kind of person they are, or were before they became ill. This is almost (but not quite) a complete waste of time. This is not to dismiss the importance of personality. In every case, one has to make an assessment of the patient's personality, and of the extent to which behaviours that are presently evident are due to illness, as opposed to personality factors. However, the assessment of personality is difficult and involves, amongst other things, an ability to infer personality characteristics from history. 'Pre-morbid' personality is a misnomer, suggesting that personality is submerged or destroyed once mental illness takes hold. This is very far from the truth. Personality remains an active shaper of behaviour even in the most severe and continuous mental illnesses, though the expression of underlying personality can be changed considerably by illness.

The main objection to this part of the history taking schema is not semantic, but practical. Hardly anyone can give an accurate account of their own personality. A remarkable proportion of anxious and troubled people will report their normal personality as 'happy-go-lucky' or even 'bubbly' in the face of evidence of chronic unhappiness. Few people understand how others experience them. No one ever describes oneself as 'insufferably pedantic' or 'touchy to the point of being paranoid', though such personalities are common enough. Assessment of personality is dealt with in Chapter 15.

The only real point in asking patients what they are like is that their answer reflects their self-esteem and their concerns about themselves. However, this is usually evident from other parts of the interview. We feel that this section should be dropped from the history taking schema altogether. Instead, in every case, an assessment of personality should stand alongside diagnosis, demanding just as much care and attention in arriving at conclusions. To leave personality assessment as a postscript to history taking seems to us to be entirely misconceived.

Main points in this chapter

1. An adequate history is the most important part of psychiatric assessment.
2. Psychiatric histories are highly structured and require the interpretation and organisation of information.
3. The standard schema of psychiatric history taking is not a guide to the structure of the interview itself.
4. History taking is never a completed task, no matter how long you have known the patient. No one can ever know everything about another human being.
5. We do not like assessment proformas or the concept of pre-morbid personality, but we strongly suspect that both of them will outlive both of us.

3

Mental state examination and psychopathology

The ability to observe and empathically understand other people is the key attribute of a good psychiatrist. It is always important to understand a patient's preoccupations, concerns and experiences. Mental state examination is a formal description of the features that are evident as the patient sits before you. The idea of mental state examination is derived from the distinction in medicine between history (the account that the patient gives of *symptoms*) and examination (looking for *signs* that can be demonstrated at the bedside). The parallel is not an exact one, as mental state examination includes exploration of experiences that are intrinsically subjective, and which may not be occurring in the here and now.

Mental state examination requires an understanding of descriptive psychopathology. This is a huge subject, much of it beyond the scope of this book. Here we explore the general principles of mental state examination. We will attempt to clarify those psychopathological issues that most commonly cause confusion.

The limitations of traditional descriptive psychopathology

Generations of British psychiatrists have been trained to follow an approach to psychopathology that is most clearly set out in Frank Fish's seminal book *Clinical Psychopathology* (Fish and Hamilton, 1985) (sadly, now out of print). However, it is apparent to most clinicians that the traditional approach is outmoded and in need of thoroughgoing revision. Although psychopathology is an important clinical tool, its limitations must be understood. Here we must issue a warning. A good knowledge of conventional psychopathology is an absolute necessity if you want to pass postgraduate psychiatric examinations. We would not want our scepticism to lead others into failure in exams that we have safely passed. Furthermore, if psychiatric training has sometimes been guilty of the reification of psychopathology as a way of understanding patients, mental nurse training frequently seriously neglects the subject.

For much of the twentieth century, psychopathologists were heavily influenced by phenomenology. This is a philosophical tool for exploring subjective experience. The idea is that it is insufficient to simply note that the patient has said something that sounds like an abnormal experience. Quite apart from anything else, variations in the ability to express oneself means that you have to be quite sure that patients are describing a bit of psychopathology rather than simply using an unusual form of words. The presence of psychiatric jargon in the general vocabulary (for example, 'I'm feeling paranoid', meaning 'I'm feeling self-conscious') makes this all the more important.

In practical terms, the phenomenologically influenced approach attempts, so to speak, to get inside the other person's head and examine the emotions and thoughts that form a mental context for each individual bit of psychopathology. Having imagined oneself into the patient's frame of mind, one can then start to explore the form and content of each idea or experience. For example, is an idea primary (arising de novo) or secondary to an emotion or another idea? Is a belief not only false, but is it also held with an abnormal resistance to reason, in which case it has a delusional level of fixity (bearing in mind that we all believe some things which are palpably not true)? Is an experience or idea understandable if you take into account the frame of mind or is it non-understandable and bizarre (in which case it may have a schizophreniform quality)? The patient's subjective experiences are compared against a set of psychopathological definitions and criteria, and then categorised accordingly.

Clearly, the approach rests on the clinician's ability to empathise and imagine. This ability is variable. Whilst it improves with experience, experience also teaches that mental experiences often do not fall into discrete typologies. For example, the definitions of delusions and obsessional thoughts are quite different, but they can mutate into each other. Some people seem to experience intermediate or mixed phenomena, and some describe experiences that seem to lie entirely outside of the standard psychopathological categories.

In recent times, CBT has been applied to a wide variety of mental disorders, including schizophrenia, and there is a growing research interest amongst clinical psychologists in psychopathology. As a consequence, a range of fundamental psychopathological concepts, such as the fixity of delusions and the non-understandability of schizophreniform symptoms, has been challenged (e.g. Garety, 1985). The increasingly articulate service user movement has forced us to critically re-evaluate many aspects of psychiatric practice, including our understanding of psychopathology. For example, 'hearing voices' probably embraces a far wider range of human experience than we previously realised (e.g. Romme and Escher, 1993).

In real clinical practice, the recognition of psychopathology can be highly dependent upon the clinician's expectations, and upon their initial assumptions about the nature of the patient's problem. For example, when uncooperative and difficult people are admitted to hospital, it is tempting to quickly decide that they are suffering from personality disorder. Their psychopathology is then interpreted through the filter of this assumption. However, a range of presentations of psychosis, from low-grade hypomania to awkward and fatuous presentations of hebephrenic schizophrenia, can look very similar. The psychopathology can only be recognised if one can distance oneself from the personality disorder assumption. Expectations always exist. One of the reasons that we emphasise hypothesising throughout this book is that it provides a way to avoid being misled by assumptions (through making them explicit and testing them).

The problem of prior assumption is equally true with regard to the recognition of phenomena that do not fit into a well-defined psychopathological type. When confronted with a conflict between what the patient says and what the textbooks say, doctors the world over have a disheartening tendency to place an unquestioning faith in textbooks. As a consequence, there is a reluctance to identify ambiguous phenomena as such, and a tendency to firmly classify them into an inappropriate category.

In the history of psychiatry, there are a number of examples of whole types of psychopathology emerging or disappearing. Whilst this may sometimes reflect real changes in the incidence of certain types of problems, it is sometimes an artefact of changing clinical fashions and expectations. For example, catatonic states were once amongst the commonest of psychotic presentations. For many years it was generally believed that such symptoms were no longer seen in the Western world, except amongst people of Asian and African origin. Fink and Taylor have strongly argued that this is not true (Fink and Taylor, 2003), but that as diagnostic fashions changed, the characteristic features of inaccessibility, mutism, posturing, overarousal and undirected excitement came to be interpreted differently.

In the light of all this, the use of psychopathology is similar to the use of diagnosis. We need descriptive psychopathology as a way of organising what we observe, but if we put faith in it as an adequate way of wholly describing our patients, it will let us down.

Doing mental state examination

There is more than one way of doing mental state examination. Finding a personal style and a range of probe questions which come naturally to the lips is more important than following a set of rules. In recent years, the use of validated instruments, such as the HAD (Zigmond and Snaith, 1983) and the KGV (Krawiecka *et al.*, 1977), has become common. Nursing staff in particular have embraced them as a useful way of exploring aspects of mental state. Like most doctors, we are instinctively rather antagonistic to questionnaires, forms and standardised instruments. Nonetheless, experience has shown that they have a role. Indeed, there are good grounds to think that they can be more effective in eliciting psychopathology than less structured approaches. They cannot, however, replace clinical skills.

Mental state examination is usually recorded following a schema like that shown in Box 3.1. This is not a guide for conducting a mental state examination. Mental state is examined throughout the interview. Psychopathology is explored opportunistically, as it arises naturally, as part of history taking, or in more informal parts of the conversation. Inexperienced and unskilled interviewers often try to conduct mental state examination as a formal exercise. They follow the schema and systematically ask questions about a large range of potential psychopathologies. As trainees, we both witnessed such interviews in ward rounds in large mental hospitals. As trainers we have watched trainees struggling to elicit psychopathology in a similar way. Patients experience this, at best, as puzzling and irrelevant, and at worst, as humiliating and anxiety provoking. It is also ineffective. Serial mental state interrogations are an extremely unreliable way of judging the progress of treatment or changes in the patient's mental health.

The best clinical interviewers approach mental state examination in a conversational and informal manner. The conversational approach relaxes the patient, who is then better able to explain their experiences. Questions that relate to the patient's concerns and daily activities are more likely to elicit psychopathologies, because this is the context in which they are experienced.

BOX 3.1 The general schema for recording mental state examination
- Appearance
- Behaviour
- Mood
- Speech
- Disorders of the form of thought
- Abnormal beliefs
- Abnormal perceptions
- Other qualitatively abnormal experiences
- Phobic symptoms
- Obsessive-compulsive symptoms
- Ideas of self-harm
- Ideas of harming others
- Cognitive testing
- Insight

In general, people suffering from anxiety or depression are readily able to describe psychopathology, as they recognise the nature of symptoms, including that they arise from within themselves. Even when depression is so severe that delusions develop, the anguish associated with the condition means that the patient wants to talk about it.

In acute schizophreniform psychosis, patients often attribute experiences that are part of their illness to the activities of others, which can create a problem in getting them to tell about the range of their experiences.

In mania, patients may not believe there is any problem at all. Milder forms of mania can be very difficult to assess in interviews. This is especially true during the recovery phase of the first episode. The patient, lacking previous experience of being unwell, finds it hard to identify remaining symptoms, and may still not recognise that they have been ill. The clinician has no experience of the patient as a person, and therefore cannot judge whether the improvement represents a return to their normal self or not. Asking disconnected questions about whether thoughts are still racing, whether they feel they have special abilities, whether they are making ill-judged decisions, and so on, are unlikely to elicit remaining problems. More fruitful is a discussion as to what they have been doing, what concerns they have, what plans they are making and how they are getting on with their family. Although it is still possible to miss residual psychopathology, this focus on the tangible and the relevant is likely to expose the way that the patient is thinking, how they have been behaving and therefore what psychopathology is still present. This general principle applies in a range of situations where psychopathology is hard to elicit.

Deciding what type of psychopathology is present can also be difficult. We have noticed over a long period of time that trainees are reluctant to ask obvious, common-sense questions. This is unfortunate, as these questions more often illuminate psychopathology than do more formal, structured questions. These questions tend to be 'What?' 'Why?' 'Who?' and 'How?' For example, 'What is it that keeps distracting your attention?', 'Why are you so tense at the moment?', 'How is it possible for people to interfere with your thoughts?', 'Why are the CIA bothering to follow you?' or even simply 'How does that work, then?' If a patient wears sunglasses throughout an interview in an ordinarily lit room, it may be in conformity to fashion, or because they have a black eye, or because they are paranoid or for some other reason. The only way of understanding is to ask why.

Sometimes it is necessary, towards the end of the interview, to ask direct questions about symptoms which may not have been mentioned earlier. What is to be avoided is asking a blitz of stereotyped questions about every potential mental state abnormality. It is possible to get suggestible people to agree that they have every symptom you mention. It is better to use probe-questions than menus of potential symptoms, and we give some examples below. To reiterate, above all it is important to help patients to explain what they are actually experiencing rather than persuading them to give a classical, but inaccurate, account of their symptoms.

On the question of note-keeping, it is normally best to write down the exact nature of any mental state abnormality as soon as you have a clear description, as details are often forgotten by the end of even brief interviews. It is no good to record that delusions and hallucinations (or any other psychopathologies) are present without writing down as much as you possibly can about the nature and content of these. You, and others, will need this information at a later time. It is best to record in as much detail as possible, and verbatim examples are especially helpful.

The only way to become skilled at mental state examination is to talk with lots of patients, not just as part of formal clinical interviews, but also informally. There is absolutely no substitute for sitting and talking over a cup of tea. Clinical interviewing can only offer a certain level of understanding of what it is like to be mentally ill. Knowing one's patients in more relaxed moments assists in developing a more profound understanding of the nature of mental illness. It helps you to see not just what is wrong, but also what is preserved; to understand the effect of mental illness on ordinary everyday activities; and to witness certain types of experiences as they actually happen, rather than through retrospective accounts. The strength of nurse training is that nurses do this all the time; one of the weaknesses of psychiatric training is that doctors tend to feel that they should remain aloof from such apparently banal activities.

Appearance and behaviour

This is generally the most neglected part of mental state examination, perhaps due to the lack of categories of abnormality in appearance and behaviour. However, the ability to observe is an absolute pre-requisite for doing mental state examination well. Observation is an active process. You have to be able to notice what is there. If appearance and behaviour are unusual, you have to be able to break the observation down into component parts and work out exactly what is not right.

Observation extends beyond spotting outlandish clothing or strange behaviour. Some years ago, a psychiatrist (one of us) interviewed a very depressed man who was unable to give much information. In a moment of drifting attention, the psychiatrist noticed that there was a blob at the end of each hair on his head, and correctly surmised that his hair had been burned. When asked how this had happened, the man explained that he saved on paying barbers by burning his hair with a match. The revelation opened up many issues about his long-term functioning and ability to care for himself.

Mood

Although attempts have been made to define a distinction between 'mood' and 'affect', for all practical purposes they mean the same thing. Mood is not a uni-dimensional emotion on a happiness–sadness spectrum, with depression and mania at the extremes and euthymia in the middle. It has a complex, multifaceted quality. Within normal experience, 'happiness' can include contentment, blissfulness, restless excitement and playfulness, each having some unique qualities. Furthermore, mood is reactive to circumstances. It modulates and changes over short periods of time, against a background of more persistent prevailing feelings. The standard psychopathological descriptions set out the major mood abnormalities (depression, elation, anxiety, anger, perplexity). These can co-exist in all combinations, including elation and depression (in the so-called mixed affective state), and depression and anger. The clinical description of mood involves recognition of the subtleties.

The identification of disorders of reactivity and modulation of mood is difficult. The most straightforward is labile, or abnormally reactive, mood. This is part of the manic syndrome, but it can occur in other circumstances. For example, people who are anxious often shift quickly from nervous giggling to tears.

The converse state, flattened affect (the loss of normal modulation and reactivity of mood) is more troublesome. We normally think of this as the emotional component of the negative symptoms of chronic schizophrenia, where it is associated with a lack of drive and volition, and with an apparent indifference to the environment. However, people who are depressed frequently show marked flattening of affect, as their misery prevents them from engaging emotionally with the outside world. Many psychotropic drugs can induce flattened affect (giving rise to the common complaint 'This stuff makes me feel like a zombie'). People with disorders on the autistic spectrum may show very little emotional modulation. Some people who are otherwise entirely normal habitually display a dour, emotionless affect, sometimes as a backdrop to a mordant wit. Each of these very different situations can give rise to a similar clinical presentation of flattened affect. Some care is needed to tell them apart.

Incongruous affect presents similar difficulties. Although there may be a variety of types of incongruous affect, in practice it almost always presents as giggling for no reason. This is a symptom of acute schizophreniform psychosis. It is especially common in hebephrenic states, which are dominated by thought disorder, perplexity and strange behaviour, with an absence of consistent and prominent delusions and hallucinations. Hebephrenia commonly occurs in adolescence. Giggling is often a response to remarks made by hallucinatory voices, in which case it is actually a congruous response to an abnormal experience. In addition to this, thought disorder and general disorganisation of mental functioning can make people see humour where others see none, and this is usually apparent when you ask them what is funny. However, every schoolteacher knows that disaffected, awkward teenagers use giggling as a defiant strategy. Some people try to control anxiety through a sort of humourless flippancy. One of the major behavioural consequences of cannabis intoxication is incongruous giggling. There are therefore a range of causes for incongruous giggling which are especially common in young people, only some of which are related to mental illness. Asking 'why?' may or may not clarify matters.

Generally speaking, abnormalities of mood are easy to detect through observation and listening throughout an interview. Changes in mood have profound effects on the minutiae of behaviour, and ordinary social interaction hinges on detecting and responding to the other person's mood. Despite this, it is important to ask people about their mood (e.g. 'What has your mood been like?') because a minority of people hide depression behind a smiling mask, which only slips in response to a direct question about their feelings.

One needs to ask about factors that provoke changes in mood. This can help distinguish the true diurnal variation of severe depression (usually worse in the morning) from diurnal patterns sustained by other factors, for example the arrival home of a partner. One should also ask about irritability and the typical precipitants for irritable outbursts. These are not always spontaneously mentioned, and they can be important in assessing the atmosphere in the household and behaviour towards family, especially children.

Where depression is present, questions about despair and hopelessness are the most reliable indicators of its severity. Probes should be aimed at establishing what the patient thinks is going to happen to them, for example 'Do you think you're likely to get better eventually?' This in turn naturally leads to questions about suicidal thoughts, for example 'Has it ever got so bad you've thought of killing yourself?' Assessment of risk is a big subject, and we deal with it in Chapter 16.

We have mentioned alterations in appetite, sleep and concentration in the previous chapter, but in the sequence of an interview, one often asks about them alongside questions about mood.

Speech and thought

One is interested in the form rather than the content of thought, hence the term 'formal thought disorder', the adjective meaning 'of form' rather than 'proper'. Thought is entirely inaccessible, and it can only be assessed through the intermediary of speech. It is important to be vigilant for speech problems when assessing whether there is formal thought disorder. Thought disorder has a high diagnostic weighting, and schizophreniform thought disorder is sometimes regarded as pathognomnic (i.e. it occurs exclusively in that disorder).

There are a number of speech disorders. The most common are subcultural inarticulacy, stuttering and dysphasia. The first of these is due to poor education, leading to both restricted vocabulary and poor self-confidence. It displays itself in muddled speech combined with difficulty in elaborating and explaining. This requires patience and encouragement from the interviewer, as it tends to improve when the person is relaxed.

Stuttering is not always obvious when the person has learned to control it. Techniques to control stuttering include pausing, looking for alternative words or altering the direction of what is being said. This can induce an odd quality to the person's speech, which can become somewhat robotic.

Dysphasia is a frequent sequela of brain injury. It often affects older people after strokes (cerebro-vascular accidents), but it is also common in younger people after closed head injuries (e.g. in road traffic accidents), sub-arachnoid haemorrhage and encephalitis. The commonest problem is in word-finding. As with stuttering, many people find an accommodation to the problem, which can make their speech sound odd. They stop and try to find a different expression, or repeatedly use the same word to stand in for words they cannot find. Some people use a stock obscenity, as such words are grammatically flexible ('Oh fuck, the fucking fucker's fucking fucked': expletive, adjective, noun, adverb and verb). This makes them seem foul-mouthed and socially disinhibited. Where a less offensive word is used, it can appear to be a neologism (see below). The possibility of dysphasia should be borne in mind wherever there is a history of head or brain injury.

In mania and hypomania, the classical descriptions of pressure of speech and flight of ideas do hold true. Everything is speeded-up and the person endlessly digresses, their ability to follow a logical thread severely compromised by punning, alliteration, rhyming, clang associations and so forth. Lesser degrees of this (so-called prolixity) is hard to assess, as similar over-inclusive, digressive thinking is commonly seen in people who are pedantic by nature, and in the habitually garrulous. Some people with very obsessional personalities are so concerned with completeness that they have to speak quickly in order to

> **BOX 3.2 Some features of schizophreniform thought disorder**
> - Concrete thinking: a failure of abstract thinking where metaphor takes on a literal quality.
> - Loosening of associations: ideas lack proper links, which gives a 'woolly' and inconclusive quality to what is said.
> - Over-inclusiveness and inter-penetration of themes: clarity of thinking is lost because too many ideas are linked together.
> - Logical failures: more severe than simple woolliness, thinking shows 'derailment' or 'knight's move' and, without acknowledgement, the train of thought alters completely. This often is related to the intrusion of a completely unrelated concept.
> - Drivelling: an unpleasant term; syntax and grammar are preserved, but thinking becomes so muddled and disorganised that the person appears to be talking for the sake of it, without conveying anything.
> - Neologisms: strictly speaking the use of an invented word to describe a phenomenon outside of ordinary experience, but more commonly the use of an existing word in an idiosyncratic and bizarre way (e.g. a patient complained of 'email', meaning thoughts inserted by other people, which he thought was due to the use of ecstasy, i.e. MDMA or 'E').
> - Word-salad: the total breakdown of all syntactical and grammatical structure where thinking becomes a series of unrelated words.

avoid their digressions being interrupted, and this can resemble hypomanic prolixity.

Schizophreniform formal thought disorder is undoubtedly a key feature of the condition, though it is far from invariable. Whilst experience improves most clinical skills, it can be an impediment to the recognition of this type of thought disorder. One comes to understand each patient's preoccupations, experiences and lifestyle. When they suffer acute relapse of psychosis, one can follow their train of thought. Years of familiarity with disordered thinking robs it of the quality of oddness, which ordinarily is the most striking feature. The only way we know of overcoming this is to try and spot the main features as a deliberate exercise. Although one rarely encounters thought disorder that exactly conforms to the classical descriptions, the discipline is helpful in detecting formal abnormalities. Some of the features are set out in Box 3.2.

Abnormal beliefs

There are a number of definitions of a delusion, which can be summarised as: 'a false and unshakeable belief, which is out of keeping with the patient's social and cultural background'. Delusions are the commonest symptom of psychosis and they generally conform to this conventional definition. The definition is, however, inadequate. Every element is subject to major exceptions (delusions can be true, they are not necessarily totally unshakeable, and other people who are not mentally ill may share similar beliefs). Furthermore, some beliefs (for example, some unusual religious beliefs) meet the criteria without being conventionally regarded as delusional. The use of the concept of the 'over-valued idea', which is applied to delusion-like ideas, only adds to the confusion. For example, people with anorexia nervosa often believe that they are fat, when objectively they are thin. This is said to be an over-valued idea, but the only reason for regarding this as anything other than a delusion is convenience. It is regarded as unhelpful and misleading to conceptualise anorexia nervosa as a psychosis. There are quite a few other problems and overlaps in addition to these, for example, the over-expansive ideas and plans of the grandiose wishful thinker, whose expectations are not strictly impossible but are extremely unlikely to come to fruition.

It would be nice to think that someone will produce an evidence-based approach to sort these problems out, but for the time being one just has to accept that there are ambiguities, and that from time to time one is bound to come across situations where it is hard to tell if someone is deluded or not. The most useful question in making the assessment is 'How do you know that?' It is in exploring the logic behind a strange belief that one comes to have some sense as to whether it is delusional or not.

Delusions are said to be either primary or secondary. Primary delusions come with a quality of sudden insight ('I suddenly knew what was happening') and are said to be unrelated to other ideas or evidence. Primary delusions are almost always preceded by a delusional mood, a strong sense that something indefinable is wrong with the external world, and the delusion carries a crystallising sense of understanding. Schneider, in delineating his first rank symptoms (Schneider, 1959) referred to delusional perception, a sudden delusional belief linked to an unrelated perception ('The television flickered and I realised my father was Satan'). In our experience, it is difficult to find these phenomena unless one interviews the patient very early in the development of the illness, possibly because they are later lost amongst other secondary symptoms.

It is always important to fully explore delusional ideas. Delusions about specific individuals in the immediate environment are quite likely to lead to action and therefore risk. For example, men with jealous delusions about their partners often act aggressively. However, it is always important to ask people what they intend to do about delusional beliefs. Even where delusions are held about remote figures, people can get into terrible trouble through acting upon them, for example by trying to contact famous people under delusions of mutual love.

When people are acutely psychotic, delusional beliefs are highly salient, which is to say they loom large in their awareness, and they are usually very bothered by them. Under these circumstances, delusions are not difficult to elicit. When psychosis is controlled by medication, or where the person has been continuously unwell for years, the ideas often persist but salience diminishes. They come to resemble unusual opinions, and they may not be mentioned spontaneously. Some people, deluded and preoccupied, nonetheless recognise that their ideas sound peculiar, or come to realise that professionals regard them as evidence of mental disorder. All of these situations can make delusions hard to elicit. We know of no general-purpose probes to deal with this. One has to probe by asking about specific ideas, and one can only find probes through informant accounts of odd ideas or prior knowledge of the patient. This seems to be universally known as 'knowing what buttons to press', as once the relevant ideas have been raised, even the most guarded people with delusions tend to talk about them freely.

Abnormal perceptions

Auditory hallucinations

By far the most common abnormal perceptions are 'voices'. They were once regarded as mainly affecting people with schizophrenia and organic cerebral problems, but it is now clear that significant numbers of people with neither problem experience them (van Os *et al.*, 2000). At present, there is no exhaustive classification of 'voices'. For example, people with borderline personality disorder often complain of hearing voices, and are sometimes thought to be either describing unpleasant thoughts or else just making it up. However, their complaints of voices are consistent, and it is a very poor principle to assume that groups of patients lie about their experiences.

A wide range of organic factors can induce hallucinations, some specific, such as high doses of amphetamines, and some non-specific, such as delirium. Some types of hallucination are clearly organic in origin, but the mechanism by which they are induced is obscure. A prominent example is alcoholic hallucinosis, which occurs after years of heavy drinking, and tends to persist through months of abstinence. The hallucinosis is mainly auditory, and arises without fixed delusions or other psychotic phenomena.

Organic hallucinations generally have a vivid, concrete and frightening quality. Where there is no clouding of consciousness, the false perceptions have the same quality as true perceptions. However, the person can readily pick up on environmental clues that they are 'hearing things'. People suffering from organic hallucinosis are particularly likely to show major behavioural responses to hallucinations. Where the person vigorously converses with hallucinations, one must always suspect an organic origin. We are always reminded of the features of organic hallucinosis by the sight of solitary alcoholic vagrants. They shout aggressively, but when approached they are usually perfectly pleasant. They will freely admit that they are shouting at voices, not because they think they are real, but because it makes them feel better. They will volunteer that the alcohol causes the voices.

Conversely, whilst people with schizophrenia are often quite certain that auditory hallucinations are real, it is clear that they have a very different quality to true perceptions. Indeed, the vast majority of people who suffer auditory hallucinations, when asked whether they hear voices, confirm that they do. Although the classical auditory hallucinations of schizophrenia are in the third person, second person auditory hallucinations are equally common. Behavioural responses to hallucinations in schizophrenia tend to be limited to pausing and listening or looking at the places where voices seem to be coming from, though active replying to voices does occur.

Traditionally, the distinction between hallucinations and non-hallucinatory 'voices' turns upon whether the experience arises within subjective or objective space. This has led to the widespread practice of asking people whether the voices arise from within their head or not. In our opinion, the use of this question is to be avoided, as it does not clarify the nature of the experience. The distinction really turns upon whether the false perception is experienced as arising from within the self or elsewhere. The self has no anatomical or geometric location. The crucial question to ask is: what does the patient think causes the voices? If the cause is entirely external, then the experience is more likely to be a hallucination, though this isn't absolute, as some people have partially self, partially non-self explanations for both types of experiences.

The content of hallucinations should be explored if one can, though many patients find it hard to clearly describe what is said. Fragmentary, derogatory hallucinations can occur in severe depression, though they are more common in schizophrenia. The diagnostic value of exploring content is not high, but it is important in understanding what the patient is experiencing. Command hallucinations are significant. These are hallucinations that instruct the patient what to do. Simply asking if the voices ever give instructions is usually sufficient to elicit them. Command hallucinations are relatively common, but a minority of patients act on them, which can create serious risks. Where there are command hallucinations, one needs to fully explore the content and the factors, if any, which restrain the person from acting.

Pseudo-hallucinations and related phenomena

There are several psychopathologies that are broadly similar to true hallucinations. It can be very hard to distinguish delusions of reference from hallucinations. Classically, delusions of reference are beliefs that neutral and impersonal materials, such as television programmes or car number plates, carry a personal and intentional message. However, patients often report that the television or other media do not allude but actually mention them by name or show pictures of them. This can be significant in distinguishing persistent delusional disorder (where there are delusions but no other psychotic phenomena) from schizophrenia (which is more likely to respond to treatment).

Obsessional ruminations are sometimes first mentioned as 'voices'. As stated earlier, some people describe symptoms intermediate between ruminations and delusions or hallucinations.

The most vexed issue is that of pseudo-hallucinations. There are a number of different definitions, and the term is a semantic nonsense, meaning 'false false perception'. In practice, the term is applied to a wide variety of experiences, and it is common for the semantic confusion to be replicated in reports that 'she's been complaining of hearing voices, but we don't think they're real voices'. Of course, *none* of the experiences that we refer to as 'voices' are objectively real. The sub-text is usually that the patient is complaining of a psychotic symptom without any other sign of psychosis, and is therefore disbelieved. It is, however, dangerous to easily leap to the conclusion that people are feigning psychotic symptoms. As a rule of thumb (based on experience), when one is 100% certain that a patient is feigning psychotic symptoms, there is a 50% chance that, in the fullness of time, they will turn out to have been mentally ill all along.

In practice, the only way that we have been able to resolve the issue of pseudo-hallucinations has been to accept that there is a heterogeneous group of experiences that are very similar to hallucinations. These either occur in the absence of any other evidence of psychosis (or cerebral disorder), or arise with a simultaneous awareness that whilst they sound 'real', they are not. They are almost invariably associated with underlying severe emotional distress. The only major exception is a small group of individuals in the general population, neither evidently mentally disordered nor distressed, who have a strong religious faith and who hear the voice of God in their everyday lives. We recognise that they may be right about the origin of the experience, but we prefer to believe that it is due to some other, as yet poorly understood, psychological process.

Non-auditory hallucinations

Hallucinations can, of course, arise in any sensory modality, and sometimes outside of the normal sensorium (for example, powerful feelings of an invisible presence). Non-auditory hallucinations in psychosis are frequently ambiguous experiences, somewhere between hallucinations, delusions and delusional misinterpretations of normal experiences, for example, the feeling of worms crawling under the skin, or of something alive in the abdomen. Visual hallucinations are more common in schizophrenia than traditional teaching has suggested (Cutting, 1990), and these are sometimes multimodality experiences (for example, demonic shadows that enter the bedroom, whose hot breath can be heard and felt against the skin).

Flashbacks

In the 1985 edition of Fish's book, the word 'flashback' doesn't even appear in the index. However, in recent years, these experiences have attracted an enormous amount of attention. The term was originally used to describe the return of symptoms of intoxication with hallucinogenic drugs (mainly LSD, but also cannabis) long after discontinuation of use of the drug. However, the term is now commonly used with respect to vivid visual images of distressing past experiences. These images are usually triggered by a trivial reminder of the past experience (a smell or a sound for example), and although they are brief, they are intensely upsetting. They were first described in PTSD, and were initially regarded as the most characteristic feature of the syndrome. Indeed, the fact that they have proven to be common in adult survivors of childhood sexual abuse has led some researchers to the view that the adult consequences of abuse are a form of PTSD (e.g. Ackerman *et al.*, 1998). However, such experiences seem to be common in the whole population. They can relate to memories that are upsetting or even just embarrassing, and we do not believe that they can be regarded as intrinsically pathological at all. The degree of emotional distress they provoke is more relevant than whether they are present or not.

Other psychotic symptoms

There are many other symptoms that can arise in psychosis, but the most important, and commonest, are passivity experiences and disorders of the possession of thought. These are Schneiderian first rank symptoms of schizophrenia, and hence carry some diagnostic significance.

The subjective quality of passivity experiences is that thoughts, actions or (rarely) emotions are literally under the control of an external agency. This is not a conclusion that the person arrives at, but is something they experience. There is usually a technological rationalisation (that this is achieved through computers or satellites), though sometimes the supernatural is blamed (demons, Satan or witchcraft). Such experiences are usually volunteered as one explores delusional beliefs. The probe 'Do you ever feel that someone else is controlling what you think?' tends not to be very helpful, as a large number of people feel that a parent, their partner or authority in general is excessively controlling. Hence a lot of people say yes, and then it can be confusing to try to disentangle the effect of everyday resentment towards an over-controlling relative from passivity experiences. Even asking 'How do they do that?' may not clarify matters. The probe 'Does anyone interfere with your thinking?' tends to work better, and will tend to elicit disorders of the possession of thought as well as passivity experiences.

The disorders of the possession of thought include hearing one's thoughts spoken out loud, thought insertion, thought withdrawal, and thought broadcasting. Although the term 'thought broadcasting' suggests that the person feels that everyone can hear their thoughts, more commonly it involves one or more specific individuals who can hear them. Like passivity experiences, this is usually rationalised in technological terms, such as the presence of implanted brain probes. There is again a potential confusion with an everyday experience, as most of us have people in our lives who can 'read' us or can 'tell what we're thinking'. Traditional probes such as 'Are your thoughts private?' or 'Are your thoughts your own?' seem to convey little meaning even to people who are experiencing thought broadcasting. The more direct question 'Do you ever feel there's telepathy going on?' seems to work better (Box 3.3).

BOX 3.3 A cautionary tale

A 35-year-old man was admitted to hospital after an unexplained and serious attempt on his own life. In the course of a 6 week admission, the only abnormality that he displayed was episodes of 'going blank' and staring at walls. These episodes happened several times a day. In interviews with the psychiatrist, he could explain neither the suicide attempt nor the 'blank' episodes. Eventually, the clinical team came to the conclusion that the presentation could be convincingly understood in terms of a dissociative state. The psychiatrist carefully explained the idea to the patient, who enthusiastically agreed that this made a lot of sense. It was decided he should go home, and he went off to make the necessary arrangements. Realising that they had not discussed plans for further treatment, the psychiatrist asked the nurses what the patient was doing, and was told he was busy phoning his father.

Eventually, the patient returned, and the psychiatrist said 'You've been phoning your father'. The patient asked how he knew this, and the psychiatrist, in a moment of inappropriate flippancy, said 'Telepathy'. The patient simply nodded. The psychiatrist found this odd, so he said 'That was a joke'. The patient replied 'Well, there's a lot of it going on!' The patient had catatonic schizophrenia. The psychiatrist, of course, was one of us.

Anxiety symptoms

Anxiety symptoms are rarely difficult to elicit, and are likely to be volunteered early in most interviews. Where they are not, there is no reason to avoid asking, 'Do you have any phobias?' and 'Have you ever had a panic attack?' as these words are part of the general vocabulary, and if the person does not understand, it is easy to explain. However, people sometimes use the terms in idiosyncratic ways, so it is important to clarify what they mean.

Phobias are, of course, incredibly common and come in an enormous variety of forms and degrees of severity. One regularly encounters unusual phobias, such as the fear of buttons or the fear of moderately severe injury. Some people have an unusual variant of social phobia where they can cope with good friends and complete strangers, but are anxious around people they know slightly. They invariably fail to attend the second interview. Phobias have two essential features: fear of a situation or thing, and avoidance. Avoidance can, however, take a number of different forms. Many people with agoraphobia go out and about when accompanied (which is avoidance of being alone in the feared situation), and many people with social phobia cope with social situations by getting very intoxicated with alcohol or cannabis first, which is a type of chemically mediated avoidance.

Panic attacks are extremely unpleasant but short-lived (though some people experience serial panic attacks). Where people report that the experience has lasted 20 min or more, it is unlikely to have been a panic attack (although, because they are so distressing, people can overestimate the duration). They are characterised by a feeling of terror, a sense of imminent death or catastrophe, and an overwhelming desire to flee. There are usually strong physiological concomitants such as palpitations and sweating. The majority of sufferers feel short of breath during an attack, and this is due to hyperventilation. A minority of people with panic attacks, however, do not hyperventilate.

Obsessions and compulsions

We have already discussed the overlap between obsessional symptoms and psychotic symptoms. Obsessional phenomena are extremely common and some people develop such symptoms when they are depressed or become anxious about a situational problem. People are often embarrassed by these symptoms, because they tend to focus on themes of contamination, violence and sexuality, so that it is often necessary to specifically ask about them. Probes about the tendency to check things excessively (for example, doors and windows at night or the gas before going out) usually work, as checking generally accompanies all other obsessional symptoms. Even when people deny checking, they usually understand the point of the question and reveal other obsessional symptoms if they are present.

Classically, obsessional thoughts are repetitive (hence 'ruminations') and distressing. They are ego dystonic (i.e. contrary to the person's wishes or values), but are unequivocally perceived as arising from within the self. They are experienced as senseless and initially they are resisted, though resistance leads to rising anxiety. Compulsions are behaviours aimed at controlling obsessions, and usually involve ritualised activities, often centred on cleaning or counting. In severe obsessive-compulsive disorder (OCD), there is usually marked avoidance, and there can be bizarre manoeuvres such as wrapping oneself in plastic to avoid contamination or chaining oneself to the bed to avoid a nocturnal act of violence. It has long been recognised, however, that no feature is invariable. This can make it very difficult to distinguish obsessional phenomena from other types of symptoms.

There are two non-psychotic phenomena which are similar to obsessions, but which are more likely to be acted upon. The first is the resisted intention. Here, the person wants to do something, usually an act of violence, but resists because of the consequences. A typical example would be the father of a rape victim, who feels fully justified in seriously assaulting the perpetrator, but is begged by his family to do nothing for fear of imprisonment. Thoughts of violence can utterly preoccupy the person, are resisted and are accompanied by severe emotional turmoil. Such revenge-driven, resisted intentions may be provoked by less understandable affronts, for example, they may be directed at blameless hospital staff who have attended the death of a loved one, or even the perpetrator of a perceived social snubbing.

Similar resisted intentions are also seen in some people who are struggling with personality-based difficulties with aggression or sexuality during the build-up to an offence.

The second type of phenomenon is compulsion-like urges. These closely correspond to the non-psychiatric usage of the word 'compulsion'. The person has a rising sense of psychological tension and feels increasingly compelled to carry out a particular act. There is resistance, but eventually the act is carried out. This initially leads to a profound sense of relief, but this in turn is often followed by feelings of self-disgust or fear of discovery. These experiences seem to arise in a range of problems with very different origins, including bulimia, repeated non-suicidal self-laceration, some types of sexual exhibitionism ('flashing') and substance misuse.

Ideas of self-harm and of harming others

Needless to say, any ideas that suggest the patient may be thinking of harming themselves or somebody else must be fully explored, including those factors that restrain them from action. Risk assessment is more fully dealt with in Chapter 16.

Insight

The idea that there is a continuum of insight from full to none, and that insight can be quantified, is simply wrong. The terms 'no insight' and 'good insight' have very little meaning, other than in indicating the extent to which the patient agrees with the psychiatrist as to what is wrong with them. As psychiatrists can be mistaken, this conveys some information about the relationship, but very little about the patient. What is more relevant is how the patient understands their situation and what they think is likely to be helpful. For example, many people with psychotic illnesses believe their delusions to be true, but readily accept efforts to help them. They often have a sophisticated understanding of how the balance of stress and medication alters the severity of symptoms. Whether this is good or poor insight is irrelevant (one could argue the case either way), but an understanding of their attitude has real practical importance.

Main points in this chapter

1. Mental state examination rests upon careful observation and listening.
2. There are some real ambiguities regarding psychopathology, but the traditional framework is a helpful guide, provided one recognises its limitations.
3. Probe-questions about psychopathology are best framed with reference to activities and ideas that are familiar to the patient. Abstract, 'technical' questions do not work very well.
4. It is important to avoid the trap whereby prior assumptions about the nature of the problem lead to a misinterpretation of what you are told.
5. Even experienced, skilled interviewers sometimes miss important psychopathology.

4

Cognitive state assessment and organic disease

No matter what one believes with regard to the usefulness of the 'medical model' in general, there is one excellent reason for the close involvement of doctors in the care of people with mental disorders. Without exception, the whole range of psychiatric disorders can be mimicked by physical disease. The effects of physical illness, and of drugs used to treat it, frequently complicate mental health problems. People with chronic mental health problems suffer from more physical ill health than the rest of the population (Joukamaa et al., 2001). Psychiatrists draw upon their background knowledge of physical medicine far more frequently than is commonly appreciated by the rest of the medical profession. Lishman's outstanding book, *Organic Psychiatry* (Lishman, 1997), is an essential purchase for all clinical psychiatrists.

Some sub-specialties, such as old-age psychiatry and neuro-psychiatry, are primarily concerned with the psychological effects of physical disease processes. However, organic factors commonly cause concern in all forms of psychiatric practice, even child psychiatry and psychotherapy, and all mental health practitioners must have the ability to recognise the possibility that physical disorder may be contributing to a problem. Whilst this may mean asking for someone else to fully evaluate physical or cognitive state, the ability to competently carry out a basic cognitive state assessment is an essential skill for everyone involved in psychiatric assessment. It is important to recognise that cognitive impairment may not be present, or may not be detectable, in all situations where physical disorder is causing psychiatric symptoms. The key to detecting organic pathology is good history-taking and careful observation. Cognitive function testing usually serves only to confirm or refute an impression that there is a cognitive deficit.

There are two major traps as far as organic disorder is concerned. The first is to accept too easily that another doctor has 'excluded' physical disease. Physical disease can rarely be definitively excluded, and the belief that a problem is 'psychiatric' can lead doctors into hasty judgements (Box 4.1).

BOX 4.1 Neurologists can be wrong

A 48-year-old woman with a past history of depression had a first episode of mania. After discharge from hospital she dropped out of follow-up, but was treated by her GP with chlorpromazine 50 mg at night. After two years, she developed writhing, athetoid movements in her right arm and neck. She was sent to see a neurologist, who gave the opinion that this was due to tardive dyskinesia. He advised discontinuation of chlorpromazine. Three weeks later she was seen by a psychiatrist, having again become hypomanic. The psychiatrist doubted the diagnosis of tardive dyskinesia, which rarely is restricted to one limb. She asked the patient how the symptoms had started. The abnormal movements had commenced in the fingers and over a few weeks spread up the whole arm to the neck. The psychiatrist feared that there was a rapidly expanding space occupying lesion in the patient's basal ganglia, and immediately admitted her for investigation. MR scanning showed multiple inflammatory lesions throughout the patient's brain, concentrated in the basal ganglia, and a diagnosis of systemic lupus erythematosus (SLE) was made. SLE probably accounted for both the mood disorder and the abnormal movements. Management proved complex, as steroids worsened the mood disorder and antipsychotics worsened the abnormal movements.

BOX 4.2 Psychiatrists can also be wrong

A 56-year-old man with hypertension and mild diabetes was referred with a 12-month history of depression. Full assessment, including cognitive testing and a range of blood tests, showed no organic explanation and he was treated unsuccessfully with antidepressants. After about a year, the psychiatrist noticed that the patient was overweight, with coarse dry hair and a gruff voice. He did everything rather ponderously. Repeat thyroid function tests showed that the results had changed from bottom of the normal range to severely hypothyroid over 12 months. The patient made an excellent recovery on thyroxin, and was remarkably forgiving of the psychiatrist, given that they both acknowledged that the features of myxoedema had been present from the outset.

The second trap is where you have looked for, and failed to find, organic disorder, but it develops (or becomes detectable) later (Box 4.2).

There is an absolute rule in psychiatry, which should never be forgotten: *the possibility of undisclosed physical disease is part of every differential diagnosis at every stage of treatment.*

The range of interactions between disease and psychiatric symptoms is very wide, but the commonest are delirium and dementia.

Delirium

Delirium (sometimes known as 'acute confusional state') is an acute event that is very common. There is a qualitative alteration in consciousness, with impairment

---

> **BOX 4.3 Main causes of delirium**
> - Non-cerebral infections (e.g. lungs, septicaemia)
> - Cerebral infections (e.g. meningitis, encephalitis)
> - Metabolic problems (e.g. electrolyte disturbance, liver failure, hypoglycaemia)
> - Drugs (e.g. intoxication or withdrawal states – especially alcohol)
> - Focal brain lesions (e.g. tumour, cerebro-vascular lesions, sub-arachnoid and sub-dural haemorrhage)
> - Diffuse cerebral problems (e.g. cerebral hypoxia, raised intracranial pressure, multiple inflammatory lesions)
> - Head injury
> - Nutritional problems (e.g. thiamine deficiency leading to Wernicke's encephalopathy)
> - Epilepsy (e.g. post-ictal confusion)

of clarity of awareness of the environment. There are specific changes in cognitive processes. Attention can be neither sustained nor shifted in the normal way. Frequently there are perceptual disturbances, accompanied by disorientation and memory impairment. The experience is always unpleasant, and is often very frightening. Both subjectively and objectively, the person seems to be living through a series of experiences that have a 'bad dream' quality. On recovery, the person's recollection of the experience is incomplete. The actual clinical presentation can vary widely and all degrees of delirium are seen, from mild and subtle to severe and obvious. No feature is invariable but agitation, hallucinations and paranoid fears are common. As a consequence, delirium can resemble psychosis. Psychiatrists working in acute hospital liaison services are frequently asked to see delirious patients, in medical and surgical wards, who are said to have 'gone psychotic'. Box 4.3 sets out a range of causes of delirium.

A key feature of delirium is that the severity of the disturbance fluctuates through the 24 hour period, and there may be periods of complete or relative lucidity. The disturbance tends to be worst at night, probably because environmental cues for orientation are more ambiguous than usual. Other circumstances that make orientation more difficult, such as poor lighting and being left alone, also tend to worsen delirium. Vivid visual hallucinations and visual misperceptions are particularly common. Delirium is not necessarily obvious, but there may be clues from the history or mental state examination (Box 4.4).

Dementia

Dementia is a generalised loss of cognitive abilities without disturbance of consciousness. There is a change in intellect, memory and personality. It is caused

---

BOX 4.4 Delirium may not be obvious

A 67-year-old widow with chronic obstructive airways disease was admitted to a psychiatric unit with a three-day history of schizophreniform symptoms. She complained that her neighbours had been loudly talking about her, accusing her of being a prostitute, and that they had been pumping a poisonous gas through the wall, which she could smell. At night she had been frightened by sensations in her vagina, which she believed were caused by the neighbours having sex with her from next door. She also complained that they had been making the pattern on her carpet swirl around in the evenings. She had been making repeated calls to the police about her neighbours, and it was this that provoked admission. Her concentration was impaired, but there were no other abnormalities on cognitive function testing. On physical examination, she was a little short of breath and there was evidence of chronic lung disease, but no acute changes were evident. The picture appeared to be typical of late onset paranoid schizophrenia.

The admitting doctor discussed the patient with the consultant psychiatrist. On the basis of the short history and the apparent swirling of the carpet pattern, the consultant wondered about delirium and suggested the patient be given oxygen prior to any other treatment. Oxygen abolished all psychotic symptoms almost immediately. The next day the patient showed obvious signs of an acute chest infection. In retrospect, it was clear that this had been developing for several days. On top of existing lung disease, it had been sufficient to cause hypoxia and delirium.

---

by a variety of coarse brain diseases, most (though not all) of which are progressive and irreversible. The commonest causes of dementia are Alzheimer's disease, cerebro-vascular disease (multi-infarct dementia) and Lewy body disease. There are many other causes, some of which are set out in Box 4.5.

Although dementia due to different diseases may show different symptom patterns and follow different courses, the different disease processes are often difficult to distinguish clinically. All psychiatrists should be able to assess whether dementia is present. Making a reliable definitive diagnosis, on the other hand, is a specialist skill. The degree of impairment on cognitive function testing does not necessarily correlate closely to the degree of functional impairment. There may be considerable variation in the degree of cognitive impairment from day-to-day or hour-to-hour.

What is cognitive function testing for?

Clinical cognitive function testing is an attempt to make an objective assessment of some cognitive functions during an ordinary clinical interview. It is a much briefer, and less reliable, process than full neuro-psychiatric assessment

---

BOX 4.5 Dementias

- Neurodegenerative diseases (e.g. Alzheimer's, Lewy Body, Pick's and Huntington's diseases)
- Cerebrovascular (e.g. multi-infarct, cranial arteritis)
- Toxic (e.g. alcohol, heavy metals)
- Nutritional (e.g. thiamine or B12 deficiency)
- Infections (e.g. HIV, CJD, syphilis)
- Structural (e.g. space occupying lesions, diffuse brain damage such as punch drunk syndrome)
- Anoxia (e.g. after cardiac or respiratory arrest)

---

or formal neuropsychological testing. It would be impractical (and not necessarily desirable) to do exhaustive testing as a matter of routine clinical practice.

Cognitive function testing is not a good screening tool, as it generates both false positives and false negatives. Generally speaking, if there is nothing in the history to suggest an organic problem, and if mental state examination has not raised a suspicion, then it is very unlikely that cognitive function testing will add anything to the assessment of the case. In reality, few experienced clinicians carry out routine cognitive function testing unless there is a reason to do so. However, there is a strong training dictum that it should always be done, and to omit it in clinical examinations is to invite failure. Furthermore, you can only become comfortable with the process, and learn the limits of 'normal', through practice. Whilst you are a trainee, it should be a routine part of a full assessment. If there is a hint of an organic problem, cognitive function testing should always be carried out.

Doing cognitive function testing

The first thing to say about people with cognitive deficits is that they do not like to be patronised any more than anyone else does. There is no reason why an old and forgetful person should fail to notice that they are being treated like an idiot. The relationship between the doctor and the patient is just as important where the patient has a cognitive deficit as in any other situation. It may be necessary to proceed more slowly, with more explanation and more repetition, but as far as possible the cognitively impaired should be treated in the same way as anybody else.

Secondly, just as mental illnesses can be mimicked by organic disease, so all types of cognitive problems can be mimicked by functional mental illness and drug side effects. Interpretation of apparent deficits on cognitive function testing should be made cautiously where the patient is very psychotic, very depressed

> **BOX 4.6 Components of consciousness (five As)**
> - Awareness: grasp, knowledge of what's going on in the environment.
> - Alertness: readiness to respond, reactivity to stimuli.
> - Arousal: overall physiological level of mental activity.
> - Attention: the ability to focus on tasks. The ability to sustain attention is concentration.
> - Awakefulness: the converse of drowsiness.

or very anxious. Unless it is essential to assess cognitive function immediately, it may be best to postpone testing.

Prior to systematic cognitive function testing, it is important to exclude impairment of consciousness. If the patient is suffering from impairment of consciousness, it is a waste of time to fully assess cognitive function, as it is bound to be impaired, and the degree of impairment will fluctuate.

Box 4.6 sets out the component parts of full consciousness. Any of these may be impaired in normal consciousness, but together the constellation implies general impairment (or clouding) of consciousness. Assessing these rests on observation and clinical judgement. Of these, only attention is amenable to formal testing (using tests of concentration).

Mini-mental state examination

The mini-mental state examination (MMSE) (Anthony *et al.*, 1982) is a validated, internationally recognised clinical screening tool for cognitive impairment. It generates a score that has some clinical significance. It can be criticised for being crude and non-specific, but it is a usable instrument for everyday purposes. It can be easily memorised by the practitioner, and it is sufficiently robust that it will suffice as a cognitive state examination in most practical situations, particularly if the doctor can follow up positive findings with more in-depth tests. The MMSE is the only part of this book that we seriously suggest might usefully be learned by rote (Box 4.7).

Further cognitive tests

Most psychiatrists develop a small battery of clinical tests that they use to test cognitive function, which supplements or extends MMSE. It is generally best to develop a relatively small number of tests that you use regularly, as this allows a clearer understanding of the range of normal and abnormal responses. The following is not a comprehensive range of neuropsychiatric tests, but, taken with

---

BOX 4.7 Mini-Mental State Examination

Add points for each correct response.

		Points
Orientation		
1. What is the?	Year?	1
	Season?	1
	Date?	1
	Month?	1
2. Where are we?	State?	1
	County?	1
	Town?	1
	Hospital?	1
	Floor?	1

Registration

3. Name three objects, taking one second to say each. Then ask patient to repeat all three. One point for each correct answer. Then repeat the answers until patient learns all three.   **3**

Attention and calculation

4. Serial sevens. One point for each correct answer up to five. Alternatively, spell WORLD backwards.   **5**

Recall

5. Ask for names of three objects learned in Q.3. One point for each correct answer.   **3**

Language

6. Point to a pencil and a watch. Have the patient name them.   **2**

7. Have the patient repeat 'No ifs, ands or buts'.   **1**

8. Have the patient follow a three-stage command: 'Take the paper in your right hand. Fold the paper in half. Place the paper on the floor'. One point for each element completed.   **3**

9. Write in large letters 'CLOSE YOUR EYES'.
Ask the patient to read and obey.   **1**

10. Have the patient write a sentence of his or her choice. Ignore spelling errors, but it should have a subject and an object, and make sense.   **1**

Visio-spatial   **1**

11. Enlarge the design below to 1.5 cm per side, and have the patient copy it (give one point if all sides and angles are preserved and if the intersecting sides form a quadrangle).   **1**

Total points:	**30**

A score of 23 in a well-educated person or a person aged less than 60 years is suggestive of cognitive impairment.

MMSE, there is sufficient here for the generalist to make an initial appraisal of cognitive impairment.

Cerebral dominance

This can be important in localising problems. Cerebral dominance usually corresponds to handedness, but sadly, not always. Footedness and dominant eye (i.e. the eye which is easier to see with on its own) can assist in assessing cerebral dominance.

Orientation

The MMSE tests of orientation suffice most of the time, but can be misleading where orientation to, say, date is not important to the patient. It can be helpful to ask about orientation to aspects of the environment that are more important to the patient, for example, the names of nursing staff or how to get to the dining room.

Speech

Specific problems with speech can make patients seem more impaired or 'confused' than they really are, and speech disorder can mimic schizophreniform thought disorder.

Problems with speech can be divided into dysphonias (disorders of voice production, often leading to hoarse or whispered speech and abnormal cough), dysarthrias (neurological or muscular disorders of co-ordination of speech, leading to slurred or indistinct speech) and dysphasias (cerebral disorders leading to problems in understanding or finding words).

Dysphonias and dysarthrias can usually be distinguished from each other, and from dysphasias, on the basis of observation during the interview. The repetition of difficult word combinations ('red lorry, yellow lorry', 'baby hippopotamus') is especially difficult in dysarthria.

There are several dysphasic syndromes, which can be broadly divided into *fluent* and *non-fluent dysphasia*. The differences between the two are evident in spontaneous speech, and are set out in Box 4.8.

Speech can be further assessed by testing repetition (the ability to repeat words and phrases, for example, 'cat', 'chair', 'the sun is shining', 'no ifs, ands or buts'), comprehension ('point to the door', 'take this piece of paper, fold it in half and place it on the chair next to you') and naming (point to a wristwatch and ask 'What is this called?'. Then ask to name strap, face, winder etc.). According to neurologists, it is possible to use the findings to localise the problem. However, in psychiatric practice, the findings are often far from clear cut.

BOX 4.8 Fluent and non-fluent dysphasia	
Fluent	Non-fluent
Normal rate	Slowed
Fluent	Faltering, with frustration
Syntax normal	Irregular and robotic
Prominent circumloculation and paraphasia	Problems finding nouns and verbs
	Perseveration
No insight	Insight

Nominal dysphasia (or anomia) is of limited value in localising problems, but is useful in screening for dominant hemisphere lesions. If a speech problem is detected, a brief assessment of reading and writing should be carried out.

Attention and concentration

The standard test of concentration is serial sevens, asking the patient to start with one hundred, subtract seven and state the answer, take seven from that and so on. The accuracy and speed of response are both relevant. The problem with this test is that it is daunting for many people, and patients often refuse to even attempt it. On the other hand, when the patient carries out the task very rapidly, it can test the doctor's own powers of concentration to destruction. Serial threes, from 20, can be used as an alternative, but, generally speaking, asking the patient to recite the months of the year backwards or to spell WORLD backwards is better tolerated and more illuminating. Letter fluency ('how many words can you think of beginning with the letter C?') and digit span (ask the patient to remember a five-figure number, then six, then seven ... but not a telephone number) are also useful. All of these tests can be affected by problems with specific functions such as dysphasia.

Memory

Everyone knows that memory impairment is a feature of dementia. Consequently, evidence of memory impairment causes considerable concern amongst patients and their families. However, memory impairment is commonly a consequence of impaired concentration, and apparently impaired memory requires careful evaluation. Patients should be warned that you are about to test memory, and encouraged to make an effort with the task. The understanding of memory is still developing and changing. Box 4.9 sets out a basic classification of memory. Those items marked with an asterisk are worth testing routinely.

BOX 4.9 Memory

Explicit memory (memories within conscious awareness)
- Short-term (lasts only a few seconds)
   *Verbal (short-term memory for spoken information)
   *Spatial (short-term memory for spatial information)
- Long-term (all other explicit memory)
   *Episodic (personally experienced events)
   *Semantic (facts)

Implicit memory (memories outside of conscious awareness)
- Conditioning (conditioned reflexes)
- Priming (unconscious cues to memory)
- Motor skills (e.g. driving a car)

Short- and long-term verbal memory are tested in the three objects test in the MMSE (Box 4.7, items 3 and 5). Remote episodic memory becomes apparent during history taking. Recent episodic memory can be tested by asking questions such as 'What is my name/job?', 'What has been in the news lately?' or 'What did you have for breakfast?' Of course, for the latter type of question to be useful, you have to have access to a reliable informant account. Questions about the news need to be relevant to the patient's interests, and it can be helpful to remain in touch with football results and the plot lines of TV soaps.

Confabulation is where the patient fills in the gaps in their episodic memory by making things up. This appears to be for their own benefit, in other words, it seems to be unconscious rather than intentional. Confabulation is traditionally associated with Korsakoff's syndrome (profound short-term memory (STM) impairment without other cognitive impairments, usually a long-term consequence of either thiamine deficiency or carbon monoxide poisoning), but it can occur in all forms of STM impairment. The false account of events is often highly plausible, and the problem may only be evident because of conflicting accounts of events and on formal memory testing. It is entirely distinct from pseudologica fantastica, the telling of highly complex lies, which is a deliberate behaviour, nearly always associated with severe personality disorder. It is seen, for example, in Munchausen syndrome.

Semantic memory is traditionally tested by a set of questions such as 'What were the dates of the first world war?', 'Who is the prime minister?' and 'What is the capital of France?' However, these questions must be adjusted for educational level and subculture. The above questions may be part of the fundamental knowledge base for a middle-class professional, but they are likely to be completely outside of the awareness of a poorly educated teenager, currently resident in a Young Offenders' Institution.

Abstract thinking

Abstract thinking is often impaired in dementia and where there is frontal lobe damage. However, it is one of the highest level cerebral functions, and many other factors can impair it, including psychosis and anxiety. It is usually only worth testing abstract thinking where an organic problem is suspected and the patient is reasonably relaxed.

The two traditional tests are proverb interpretation and similarities/differences. Proverb interpretation is the less useful of the two. A very large proportion of the population, when asked 'What do people mean when they say "people who live in glass houses shouldn't throw stones"?' reply, 'Well, they'll break the windows'. It can be surprisingly difficult to judge the degree of abstraction involved in a specific answer. In any case, proverbs are culture bound, and potentially misleading when applied to people from ethnic minorities. The proverb most commonly used in this test is 'Too many cooks spoil the broth'.

Similarities/differences is altogether more useful. The patient is asked 'What are the similarities between a chair and a table?' and 'What are the differences between a child and a dwarf?' Normal answers depend on recognition of categorical similarities and differences, rather than concrete features such as 'They both have four legs'.

Judgement

Judgement is really a specific aspect of abstract thought. Impaired judgement is obvious and alarming to those around the patient, but it is hard to test clinically. The patient is normally unaware of it. Consequently, it is most easily assessed through the history given by family and friends. The usual clinical test is to give the patient a scenario involving a judgement and asking them what they would do, for example, 'You are in a cinema and you notice that a discarded cigarette has started a small fire'. The assessment of the patient's response is subjective, and it is best to be cautious about the reliability of this kind of test, unless the response is grossly abnormal.

Parietal lobe tests

The dominant and non-dominant parietal lobes have different functions. Dominant parietal lobe functions can be tested more reliably than non-dominant.

The overlapping pentagons test in the MMSE (Box 4.7, item 11) tests for constructional dyspraxia, which is a dominant parietal lobe sign. The patient can also be asked to draw a house. An oversimplified drawing indicates a dominant lesion; an exploded drawing may be due to a non-dominant lesion.

Box 4.10 sets out some more specific parietal lobe tests.

BOX 4.10 Parietal lobe tests

Dominant parietal lobe tests

- Finger agnosia: Ask the patient to name which finger you touched. Touch two fingers on each side.
- Left–right disorientation: Ask the patient to put their right hand on the desk, then remove it. Repeat with left hand, then right hand again.
- Praxis: Ask the patient to mime how they would comb their hair, use scissors, clean their teeth, blow out a match. Watch for inability to do these and also for use of body parts as objects (e.g. cleans teeth with a finger).
- Calculation: Ask patient to write down five numbers and add them up.
- Writing: Ask patient to write a sentence.

Non-dominant parietal lobe tests

- Postural arm drift: Ask patient to hold out the arms, palms down, eyes closed. Watch for drift of either hand downwards. Arm drift indicates contralateral parietal lobe abnormality.
- Unilateral neglect: Ask patient, eyes closed, to tell you which hand you touched. Touch left, right, both together.

Frontal lobe tests

Box 4.11 sets out some reliable tests for frontal lobe dysfunction, but they are relatively insensitive, which is to say, the dysfunction has to be severe before the test becomes abnormal.

Perseveration is a frontal lobe sign, which can manifest itself either in speech or in behaviour, and consists of inappropriate repetition. The person seems unable to shift to a new frame of reference. At one end of the spectrum it may involve the repetitive use of a word far beyond its meaning (for example, an 80-year-old man from Benfleet, Essex, who, in reply to direct questions, said he had fought in Benfleet during World War II and that he smoked Benfleet cigarettes), and, at the other end of the spectrum, may manifest itself as continual repetition of complex behaviours such as shopping, such that the patient's house fills up with decomposing groceries. Like many other signs, it may be more obvious from the history, or in conversation, than on formal testing.

Catastrophic reactions

The range of cognitive tests described here is quite daunting. Some patients, struggling to cope with cognitive tests, suddenly become very distressed or angry. This ends the interview in most cases, and also affects the patient's relationship with the doctor. It is not always possible to spot a catastrophic reaction developing. Reassurance and an awareness of the patient's reaction to poor

> **BOX 4.11 Frontal lobe tests**
> - Grasp reflex: Test by stroking both the patient's palms. An abnormal response is a reflex grasp of the stroking fingers.
> - Motor sequencing: Test by asking the patient to watch what you do and copy. Then, with arms outstretched, palms down, alternate opening and closing fists, so that, as one fist opens the other closes. Alternatively, use the Luria test: tap on the desk in a repeating sequence of closed fist on desk, edge of open hand on desk, palm down on desk. Repeat Fist, Edge, Palm several times and ask patient to copy.
> - Perseveration: Ask patient to tap three times on the table with their middle finger.
> - Alternating frames of reference: Ask patient to tap once on the table when you tap once. Then to tap twice when you tap twice. Then to tap twice when you tap once. Then to tap once when you tap twice.

performance (or sometimes to the process of being tested at all) is important. The risk of a catastrophic reaction dictates that cognitive testing usually is best conducted towards the end of the interview.

Main points in this chapter

1. All psychiatric disorders can be mimicked by physical problems.
2. An awareness of the patient's experience of the interview is just as important with the cognitively impaired as with anybody else.
3. History taking and observation throughout the interview are more important in assessing cognitive problems than formal clinical tests.
4. Psychiatric illness impairs performance in cognitive tests.
5. It is worth learning the Mini-Mental State Examination and a few other reliable cognitive tests. These should be practiced regularly.

Part II

The main principles of one-to-one interviewing

In the UK, one-to-one interviewing is no longer the dominant model of interaction between psychiatrists and patients. Psychiatrists increasingly work as part of multi-disciplinary teams, away from the traditional office setting. Supporting and supervising other professionals is becoming as important as face-to-face contact with patients. Nonetheless, the core skills of a psychiatrist are based upon the ability to work one-to-one, and many important issues are most easily understood in the office interview setting.

This section deals with some key principles and concepts through exploration of the one-to-one interview.

5

Office-based psychiatric assessment

It is said that in football, everything is complicated by the presence of the opposing team. A very similar principle applies in clinical interviews. The technical tasks outlined in Part I are quite complicated in themselves, but what really makes the situation demanding is the presence of the patient, who is likely to have unpredictable expectations and needs.

There are some key tasks that have to be carried out in any successful assessment interview. Firstly, and perhaps most importantly, the psychiatrist has to establish the foundations of a relationship with the patient. It is self-evident that a good relationship with the patient is desirable, and that symptom relief (let alone recovery) is unlikely against the backdrop of a poor relationship. What is less obvious is the exact nature of a good relationship, as it does not necessarily involve doing everything the patient wants.

Secondly, a large amount of historical information has to be collected and organised, whilst carefully observing the patient and carrying out a mental state examination.

Thirdly, the psychiatrist must arrive at both a diagnosis and a thorough understanding of the patient's problems and the context within which they have arisen. This includes an assessment of risk.

Fourthly, all of this has to be explained to the patient in a form that they can understand.

Finally, the psychiatrist has to decide what interventions are likely to be helpful, negotiate a treatment plan with the patient, and persuade them to follow it.

Fortunately, these tasks overlap with each other. In forming a relationship with the patient, the psychiatrist learns something about their social interactions. The process of assessment can have a powerful, though non-specific, impact in relieving the patient's distress.

Like driving a motor vehicle for the first time on the road, initially everything seems frighteningly complex. Before very long, multiple tasks are effortlessly carried out simultaneously. Or at least, this is how it is most of the time.

In trying to understand what goes on between psychiatrists and their patients, it is helpful to think about the different agendas each brings to the interview, and how the conflicting demands of these agendas can be resolved.

Dr Coltrane and Mrs Mitchell

Let us take the example of Dr Coltrane, an experienced psychiatrist, who is asked by a general practitioner (GP) to assess Mrs Mitchell. The referral letter states that Mrs Mitchell is anxious and depressed and that she has expressed suicidal ideas.

Mrs Mitchell

Mrs Mitchell is 40 years old, and she is very unhappy. She is irritable and she has been shouting at her family a lot. Sometimes, she bursts into tears for no reason. She is constantly tired but she cannot sleep at night. She has stopped going out with her friends, and the house is a mess. Her husband is fed up with trying to find out what is wrong with her. One evening they have an argument. Mrs Mitchell ends up in tears, and, in a mood of self-recrimination, says that the family would be better off if she killed herself. Her husband is alarmed and insists that she makes an appointment with their general practitioner.

After a sympathetic though brief chat, her GP prescribes an antidepressant. Mrs Mitchell has read about the addictive effects of such drugs, and she throws the tablets away after a few days. On returning to the GP a few weeks later, she sobs uncontrollably. She tells him about her suicidal thoughts. He suggests that it might be helpful to see a psychiatrist, and she tearfully acquiesces to the idea. Although she does not say so, she is alarmed by the suggestion. On the day of the appointment, she does not want to attend. Her husband loses his temper and angrily tells her that she is going mental and needs sorting out, before she sends him mental as well. With great reluctance, she keeps the appointment.

All interviews between doctors and patients are skewed and follow rules that are very different from other types of interactions. Ordinary social reciprocity is suspended. Doctors are permitted to behave in unusual ways and to ask intrusive questions on the understanding that the relationship has a primary orientation towards the patient's needs, physical or emotional. This one-sided nature imparts much to the therapeutic potency of the relationship, but also has a darker aspect. There is steep power-gradient between a doctor and a patient. Even the most articulate, well-informed patient (for example, a doctor seeing his own GP) is at a disadvantage because of this power imbalance. Patients are very aware of this, which accounts for a lot of the defensive and awkward behaviour that doctors dislike so much. It is hard for doctors to stay in touch with the stressful quality of medical interviews, because they spend so much of their time in them, and they become banal. It is easy to lose sight of the fact that, whilst the doctor knows exactly how an interview is likely to proceed, many patients do not know what to expect, have little control over the situation, and so become intensely anxious. The preconceptions that patients bring to their first interview with a psychiatrist exacerbate this considerably.

Preconceptions

Psychiatrists (with a few unfortunate exceptions) are well aware that they are ordinary people, with no special insights into the human condition. The general population, on the other hand, tend to experience psychiatrists as very unusual people. Mrs Mitchell has never met a psychiatrist before, but, like everyone else, she has heard jokes, seen films and read newspaper stories. Even to broadsheet journalists, psychiatrists are indistinctly distinguished from psychoanalysts, psychologists and psychotherapists. Popular images of psychiatrists tend to fall into two types, the inept bleeding-heart liberal and the sinister all-seeing malefactor. Both stereotypes carry an implication that psychiatrists are personally suffering from a covert madness. These are powerful and frightening images.

The popular images are probably not just the consequence of a persistently bad press. Compared with other people, psychiatrists do have a real ability to penetrate the mind, to seek out people's most private fears and to detect weaknesses and insanity. On meeting a psychiatrist for the first time, either socially or professionally, many people will express this fear quite directly. This usually takes the form of a nervous joke on the theme 'I suppose you can read my inner thoughts'. Realistically, psychiatrists do have considerable legal powers to interfere in their patient's life. Most patients have no way of judging whether a psychiatrist will regard them as in need of compulsory admission to hospital. Community-based psychiatry is still relatively new, only emerging on a significant scale in the 1980s. For many ordinary people, the image of the forbidding asylum is very much alive, and with it the fear of indefinite incarceration. It is easy to understand why many patients approach psychiatrists for the first time with great anxiety. Often only desperation or duress drives them to attend their appointment.

The psychiatric mystique does have a few redeeming features. It gives the initial interview an impact beyond the routine medical appointment. The interview is likely to have a watershed quality. This can reinforce helpful aspects of the interaction, though equally, if one is insensitive to the patient's fears, the experience can prove anxiety provoking and unhelpful.

Sitting in the waiting room, Mrs Mitchell would not be able to explain why she feels so anxious, but she is unclear as to what will take place in the interview, and she has no great certainty that it will be helpful.

Agendas

A psychiatrist's and a patient's agendas at the start of an interview each include items that are explicit and items that are implicit. A patient's list of questions about medication is an example of an explicit agenda item. If the patient leaves the clinic without having tackled those matters that were important to her at the beginning of the interview, it is certain she will feel unsatisfied. She will probably feel that she has not been understood and that this doctor is unlikely to help her. She may well not come back for follow-up appointments. On the other hand, a doctor's need for the patient to like him is an example of an implicit (and even perhaps unconscious) agenda item.

Ultimately, it is the psychiatrist's responsibility to control the interview so that the patient is likely to benefit from it. Consequently, it is inevitable that his agenda is dominant. However, both agendas create legitimate demands within the interview. It certainly is not possible to simply clarify each agenda at the outset in a straightforward way. Resolving the tension caused by the differences between the separate agendas is not necessarily difficult, but it does require an awareness that such agendas exist.

Mrs Mitchell's agenda

Clearly, any individual patient's agenda is idiosyncratic, but there are themes that are common. In Mrs Mitchell's case:
1. She is worried that she might be going mad. Her current feelings and behaviour are out of character, and she cannot understand what is happening to her. Her husband and her GP both seem to think that she has a mental problem.
2. There are some behaviours that are particularly worrying her. She is very bothered by her inability to sleep. Her constant shouting at the children makes her feel badly about herself. Sometimes she worries that she could completely lose control and assault them. She has thoughts that everyone would be better off if she killed herself, and the prospect of simply not feeling anything is attractive. She knows that her suicide would be very painful for her family, but she worries that the urge might overwhelm her.
3. There are some matters that she actively wishes to conceal from the psychiatrist. The family receives state benefit payments, but both she and her

husband do casual work to supplement this. Although the sums of money are small, this is illegal and there is a well-publicised agency that investigates benefit fraud. The family needs the extra money, but she feels guilty about breaking the law, and she is fearful of the shame of being discovered. On top of this, she has guilty feelings and regrets over a termination of pregnancy in her teens. Both of these guilty secrets are relevant to her current distress.

4. She wants the psychiatrist to explain what is wrong with her. This is not the same as being given a diagnosis. When her GP told her that she was depressed, this conveyed little information to her. She has felt 'depressed' before, but her present condition is quite different and a lot worse. The concept of a depressive illness is not familiar to her. She needs an explanation in terms that she can understand and accept.

5. In addition to an explanation, she wants a plan of help that makes sense to her. Just as the explanation of what is wrong must be plausible in her terms, the treatment plan must seem credible to her.

6. Above all, she wishes to avoid adverse consequences, such as hospitalisation or the removal of her children from her care.

Dr Coltrane's agenda

The psychiatrist's agenda is not necessarily any more straightforward than the patient's:

1. He has an initial hypothesis about Mrs Mitchell's problem, based upon the GP's letter. He wants to test and elaborate this hypothesis.

2. He wants to complete the five tasks set out at the beginning of this chapter. Ideally, he wants this all completed in the first interview, so that there are no awkward loose ends to sort out later.

3. He wants to achieve this within a specific time frame, because running late has consequences for other people, makes him feel stressed, and can lead to him missing his lunch. As patients sometimes want to talk about matters that he thinks are off the point, he wants to control the interview.

4. He is curious about the patient and wants her to leave the interview feeling that he has helped her. If Dr Coltrane did not have such motivations, he would not want to work as a psychiatrist.

5. He wants to make sure that it is very unlikely that the patient will go on to do something untoward, such as harming herself or someone else. Such an event would affect his professional self-esteem, but it would also have more tangible consequences, as he would be likely to be called to account for his assessment and decisions.

6. He wants to protect himself emotionally. He works with distressed people every day, and he must remain empathetic without becoming distressed himself. Distress is infectious and sometimes patients' problems resonate with problems in Dr Coltrane's life. He wants to preserve a proper professional distance between the patient and himself. He wants to avoid making disclosures about himself or being drawn into an overly friendly relationship. These issues of boundary setting are dealt with in the next chapter.

A basic interview framework

Being a skilled interviewer involves a lot more than the use of a set of behavioural procedures. There are many different ways of conducting a good interview. Everyone has their own style, determined by their personality and modified by expertise and experience. There is no script for a perfect interview. However, the behavioural procedures, which are simple and quite well-known, are very useful. Interviews move between distinct phases. An awareness of these basics facilitates the interview, and the reconciliation of agendas.

Before the interview

Even before the interview starts, the doctor will have formed an impression of the likely nature of the problem, based on the referral letter. Over time, psychiatrists become increasingly skilled at spotting patterns and gleaning information from such letters, despite the fact that they are often brief. You learn about the micro-demography of the area that you work in, and the likely life-style of people living in particular streets. One learns what types of patients are drawn to individual GPs, and the types of referral that each GP tends to make. Taken alongside age, gender and the main symptoms, a preliminary guess about the nature of the problem is more likely to be right than wrong. Such assumptions are likely to be present, whether or not one makes them explicit. This immediately creates a trap. Unless these assumptions are formed into an explicit hypothesis that can be tested and pursued, initial assumptions can undermine the objectivity of the assessment, and they can drive a process whereby you find what you are looking for and fail to spot that which you do not expect. Hypothesising starts before the interview. The psychiatrist explicitly states to himself what he expects to find.

There is a second pre-interview discipline that is helpful in a wide variety of circumstances. This is to be clear why you are seeing the patient and what this particular interview is for. The question may seem inane, but patients are referred for a variety of reasons. This process is especially important when working in teams and in follow-up appointments, but also has usefulness in assessment interviews. For example, are you providing an opinion or deciding whether to take the patient on for treatment? Do the patient and the referrer have the same expectation of the assessment process? If you assume that, for example, all assessment interviews necessarily lead to follow-up until the point of recovery, clinics will contain a significant number of compliant but puzzled patients who do not want, or need, to be seen.

Office layout is worth thinking about, though offices are often shared and have multiple functions. Interviewing across a desk is intimidating, and it is better to have the patient at the side of the desk. Chairs should, wherever possible, be at the same height. Armchairs create informality, but they tend to be low, and can cause problems to older people and those with physical disabilities. The doctor should be able to escape from the room unimpeded and have the means to raise the alarm if necessary (these measures are very rarely needed, but when they are, they are very important). Other staff should know whether interruptions are permitted or not.

Introductions

Introductions are a courtesy that most people recognise as important in social or business settings. Unfortunately, doctors often neglect them in their work. This is a serious error. If the start of the meeting is socially gauche, the patient is unlikely to feel comfortable in talking freely about sensitive and private matters.

Dr Coltrane goes to the waiting room, introduces himself by name and invites Mrs Mitchell to his office. He could ask the receptionist to send the patient in, but a more personal approach is less intimidating. If the opportunity arises, shaking hands with the patient is a good idea. In British culture, failing to shake hands on first meeting can carry an arrogant implication about relative social status. Shaking hands, on the other hand, implies that you are taking the other person seriously. Unfortunately, there is a critical moment for handshakes, after which it becomes unhelpfully awkward, and the moment is easily missed.

Once alone in the office, a few moments devoted to social ritual give the patient the opportunity to adjust to the setting and to the doctor as a person. Dr Coltrane indicates which chair Mrs Mitchell should sit on. He closes the door. The doctor may know that the interview will not be overheard if the door is left ajar, but the patient cannot be certain of this. He explains that he is a consultant psychiatrist and that he is seeing her at her GP's request. In other words, he makes clear his profession, his status and why he's seeing her. Even in the twenty-first century, patients still arrive in psychiatrists' clinics unaware of these basic facts, and it is as well to be unambiguous before the interview starts. The patient who thinks he/she has been referred to a chest physician for breathlessness, rather than to a psychiatrist for panic attacks, and who realises this half way through the interview, is likely to be difficult to help.

Dr Coltrane explains that the interview will last about one hour. This is a long time for a medical interview, and patients often expect something much shorter. If Mrs Mitchell has later commitments, for example, if she has to pick up the children from school, the interview will start to go wrong as she realises that time is running short. A few patients think that the interview has no time limits. In either case, it is better that there is clarity about the timescale at the outset.

Helping the patient to describe their problem

Generally speaking, a good starting point is to tell the patient what you already know from the referrer. This gives the patient a point of reference as to what you need to be told, and, if they think the referrer has misunderstood, an early opportunity to say so. This is usually an exercise in précis. Simply reading out the letter, with its jargon, is generally to be avoided. 'Your GP thinks you might be psychotic' is not a good start to an interview, but 'your GP is worried about the trouble with your neighbours' is less alarming and conveys a similar meaning. There are very few good reasons not to be frank with patients, but translation from medical to English eases communication considerably.

Dr Coltrane explains what he knows, and says 'tell me about the problem'. He allows the patient to talk. He chooses not to make notes during the first part of the interview, remaining fully attentive until the general nature of the problem has become clear. Clinical note taking can be intrusive and some patients are perturbed by it. However, the practice of writing notes after the interview has finished is time consuming and invites lapses of memory. At some point in the interview, one must start making notes. It can be helpful to explain, for example, 'I'm going to write down what you've told me, so that I don't forget'. If the patient is sensitive about confidentiality and record keeping, this creates an opportunity for them to raise their concerns, and in any case makes it clear why the notes are kept and that the information is being taken seriously.

The psychiatrist's comments in the early, unstructured, part of the interview need to be fairly neutral and aimed at helping the patient to express herself. For example, Mrs Mitchell weeps and hesitates as she describes her irritability, how she shouts at the children and how they become upset. There are a number of clichéd stock phrases used by generations of psychiatrists, which continue to work in helping patients to talk about difficult matters, for example:

'it's ok to cry'
'that sounds very difficult'
'that seems to be worrying you'
'take your time telling me about it'.

Similarly, if the patient cries, the offer of a box of tissues acknowledges the patient's distress, without implying that the doctor cannot cope with it. It is a mistake to try and stop the patient from crying or being upset, as this will lead the interview away from important material.

If the patient is not expressing herself clearly, it is possible to clarify without becoming prematurely directive:

Dr Coltrane: 'Can I just check I've understood this correctly? Things were ok until about nine months ago, around the time your friend was diagnosed with cancer. Things got worse in March when you had a sudden feeling that you were about to die when you were out shopping. After that you became generally more tense and anxious, and you started sleeping badly. More recently you've become tearful and very low in mood'.

This is a capsule summary, organising and feeding back part of the story. If the doctor has it right, the interview can move on and the patient knows she has been heard. If it is wrong, the patient can correct the summary. In either case, the patient knows that the doctor is taking the trouble to understand properly.

The length of the initial, unstructured, part of the interview depends upon whether one feels that cogent information is emerging. Occasionally, a patient will give a full and well-organised history spontaneously. This is rare. Most people, when talking about themselves, will eventually wander and start to interdigitate themes. This is hard for the listener to follow (we have all had this experience when cornered at parties). At this point, the doctor must intervene.

Hypothesis testing

By now, the psychiatrist will either have a more complicated version of his initial hypothesis or a completely new hypothesis about the nature of the problem. The next, more directive, phase of the interview aims to both test the hypothesis and to fill out the overall picture. This means asking about symptoms that have not been volunteered: both symptoms that are normally expected, in keeping with the hypothesis (in Mrs Mitchell's case loss of appetite, diurnal variation of mood, impaired concentration etc.) and symptoms associated with alternative explanations (in Mrs Mitchell's case, long-standing phobic symptoms and obsessional symptoms). Throughout, Dr Coltrane attempts to relate symptoms to antecedents, for example by asking about stresses in Mrs Mitchell's life at the time of the onset of symptoms. He asks about alterations in behaviour consequent upon the symptoms.

Mrs Mitchell is tearful and distressed. She feels that the problem started when a close friend was diagnosed with cancer nine months earlier, but that things had become much more difficult following an initial panic attack three months later. She has had these episodes regularly since, and has become increasingly distressed, irritable and sleepless. She is fearful that she is going mad. Dr Coltrane has established through direct questions that Mrs Mitchell was already experiencing depressive symptoms prior to the onset of panic attacks, and that these are typical hyperventilatory episodes. They have continued at a rate of about three a week, with no particular precipitants, and in no particular situation. There is no true phobic avoidance, but she has generally withdrawn from her normal activities and lacks motivation. There has been a steady worsening of depressive symptoms, including tearfulness, hopelessness, sleep disturbance (waking through the night and early waking), irritability, impaired concentration with secondary forgetfulness, loss of energy, loss of motivation and loss of libido. She has a reduced appetite, and she has lost about 5 kg weight. She frequently thinks of death and is concerned that she might take her own life, but she does not want to die. Her forgetfulness has led her to worry that she might have Alzheimer's disease like her grandmother.

In this case, the general nature of the problem matches Dr Coltrane's initial hypothesis, but the context and antecedents have yet to be fully explored.

Controlling the interview

Although interviews become increasingly structured as they proceed, the need to control the interview can arise at any stage. At the simplest, digressions and repetitions must be controlled. Clarifications are necessary, and, later on, some topics can only be dealt with through direct and closed questions. As the psychiatrist fills out the history, he has to move discussion smoothly through a range of topics, which may not appear to the patient to be logically connected. It is easy to get the degree of control wrong. Pushing the interview on too quickly can appear dismissive, and risks overlooking important information. Lack of control, for fear of causing offence, leads to an unfocused interview, which also risks omissions.

Curtailing discussion is best done explicitly, and the degree of bluntness needed depends on the patient's responsiveness to social cues:

'OK, I'd like to move on to ask you about …'
'This is obviously important to you, but there are some other things I need to understand'
'We seem to have drifted off the point. Let's go back to what you said about …'
'Hang on, STOP, I've lost track here. Tell me about …'

These remarks vary in subtlety, but all are polite and signal a clear intent. Only very occasionally does the doctor have to give up and let the interview go where it will, usually with the need to bring the patient back for a second interview in order to gain more coherent information.

It is considerably easier to stop patients from talking than it is to get them to talk when they are reluctant to do so. Where a patient is hesitant, or obviously distressed, on being asked about a particular area of their life, it is usually helpful to acknowledge this. A comment such as 'you look really uncomfortable' followed by silence can allow the patient to approach the difficulty more gradually. The process of drawing out emotionally charged information from someone has more to do with not allowing the subject to change than it has to do with questioning per se. If it becomes apparent that the patient really does not want to discuss something, one can attempt to defuse the situation and gain some information by a (somewhat disingenuous) ploy such as 'Look, you are obviously very uncomfortable with this, so don't tell me about it. Just tell me why this is difficult for you'.

A major strategy we all use to avoid emotionally laden subjects is vagueness. Vague answers to important questions demand the use of tightly closed questions and an emphasis on specifics:

'When does *x* happen?'
'Tell me about the last time that happened'
'What did you do next?'
'Ok, how much did you drink yesterday?'

Non-verbal communication

Within an interview, non-verbal communication is important, both in assessing the patient and as a tool for the doctor. Patients communicate their state of ease or distress in the here and now mainly non-verbally, for example by facial expression, by maintaining or avoiding eye contact, by adopting different postures and so on. Because all communication is reciprocal, the doctor automatically responds non-verbally (or appears robotic if he does not). Attention to the patient's non-verbal behaviour is part of mental state examination, but it also reflects how the patient experiences the interview. The tense, uneasy patient needs more social introduction at the start of the interview than someone who is obviously more composed. Non-verbal cues signal the affect associated with different subjects and may mark areas where the patient has significant problems, but has difficulty in saying so.

There are some non-verbal tools at the interviewer's disposal that can be used to control the interview. They are, principally, gestures aimed at encouraging the patient to talk, gestures aimed at holding close attention on a particular subject, and those aimed at closing off a particular subject. The gestures are familiar from ordinary social intercourse. One's skill in using them professionally largely depends on possession of the corresponding social skills in ordinary life (although, like many other things, this can sometimes be faked).

Encouraging the patient to talk freely rests on an impression of interest and an illusion of unhurriedness. Gestures therefore indicate that the doctor is relaxed, for example, moving back from the desk and adopting an 'open' body posture. Discarding the case notes temporarily and with some deliberation, though quasi-theatrical, can give a message of particular attention. This type of manoeuvre allows the maintenance of eye contact.

Holding attention on a particular topic involves further gestures of attention. Abandonment of the case notes and close eye contact apply here too, though open body postures are less useful. On the contrary, leaning forward and refusing to relax a body posture discourages a shift away from the subject. This may involve overriding the patient's body language of discomfort. It is a fine judgement how far to sustain this. If overdone, it can create the appearance of a maniacally staring-eyed, hunched psychiatrist, which may confirm the patient's worst fears.

'Closing off' gestures may be the converse of the above, or may involve a more positive and deliberate action. Picking up the case notes again indicates an alteration in the interview, as does reversion to a closed posture. Winding up or summarising comments are usefully accompanied by corresponding hand movements. An open palmed gesture is a clear signal to stop.

The structured part of the interview

Very few people have a clear understanding of the way in which contextual factors provoke and shape their mental illness. Drawing out this narrative is a powerful, but non-specific, therapeutic factor in psychiatric interviewing. By moving systematically through the standard structure of the psychiatric history (set out in Chapter 3), contextual factors become apparent. If the relationship between patient and psychiatrist is developing satisfactorily, then issues that the patient never intended to mention, such as Mrs Mitchell's worries over benefit fraud, may be disclosed. Essentially, the patient decides that the psychiatrist is trustworthy. Even where difficult material is not immediately volunteered, there are often clues in the history or in the patient's response to particular types of questions. Attentiveness to clues, gaps and bits of history that do not make sense is what allows psychiatrists to uncover the most difficult parts of patients' stories.

Recording the history as a time line, a strict chronology, will reveal relationships between events. Gaps in the chronology should be explored, as they can mark important secrets, such as periods of imprisonment.

Current preoccupations can offer clues to important past events. Mrs Mitchell's guilt over benefits, and fear of loss with respect to her friend, both have a thematic link with her unresolved feelings over the termination of pregnancy. Questions about other things that make her feel guilty or (alternatively) other difficult losses in her life may well lead to a disclosure.

There is a caveat here. Forced disclosure is not a legitimate part of an assessment interview, and it requires a fine judgement to decide how hard to push patients on issues that distress them. It can be tempting to guess what lies behind a patient's distress, and to put the guess to them. This is not a good idea, as patients sometimes agree to suggested histories that are not correct and, in extreme cases, may sometimes be persuaded of their veracity.

By working his way through the history, and completing those relevant parts of mental state examination omitted earlier, Dr Coltrane comes to an initial assessment of Mrs Mitchell's problem. This is still a hypothesis, because the process of hypothesising is never truly completed. New information can always emerge, and one becomes incrementally more certain, but never unshakably so.

Mrs Mitchell is a woman with an anxious, perfectionist personality. She is religious, and has high moral expectations of herself. She had a termination of pregnancy in her teens, which is the subject of continuing guilt. Her best friend had a hysterectomy for cervical carcinoma nine months ago, and Mrs Mitchell worries that she will die. She has become increasingly concerned about her own health. The couple have debts, which is why they take casual work. Forgetfulness and the onset of panic attacks exacerbated her fears over physical health, and rising anxiety provoked further panic. Her anxiety, depression and irritability have led to a deterioration in her marriage, making her feel worse about herself, and hence more depressed. She worries that she may hit the children and that they may be taken out of her care. She also worries that she will take her own life, and that the children's lives will be blighted.

No single factor has directly caused her current misery, but when taken together in the context of her life, it is understandable how these stresses have come together at this time with a consequent reaction of a moderately severe depression with secondary anxiety.

Reassurance

Some of Mrs Mitchell's initial agenda items invite a response of reassurance. Her fear that she has dementia was raised early on. Towards the end of the interview, Dr Coltrane had sufficient history to firmly decide that her forgetfulness was due to impaired concentration. He could then truthfully reassure her.

Not all such fears are so easily dealt with. Mrs Mitchell's fear of hospitalisation was expressed early in the interview. Dr Coltrane already knew that it was unlikely that he would want to admit her, but it was too soon to be sure. Similarly, later on, her fear of the involvement of child protection agencies could not be immediately dealt with. It is very tempting to offer reassurance on these kinds of issues, but it is essential to be truthful. A qualified reassurance will heighten rather than relieve anxieties ('Your children will probably not get taken away'). The habit of premature reassurance inevitably leads eventually to a betrayal. Someone will eventually prove to pose a higher risk than one initially supposed. All that the psychiatrist can do is to acknowledge the patient's anxiety, and promise to return to the subject at the end of the interview. There is a real dilemma over how much reassurance to give, and if in doubt, it is best to explicitly delay the question till the end of the assessment.

Closing the interview

Interviews need proper endings. Hopefully, the movement between free discussion and direct questioning, giving feedback through capsule summaries, the systematic exploration of context and attentiveness to clues would have allowed Dr Coltrane to deal with his own agenda whilst allowing Mrs Mitchell to disclose hers. However, at the end of the interview, Dr Coltrane checks that Mrs Mitchell does not hold undisclosed information or agenda items. The closing question, 'Is there anything else that you feel it is important for me to know?' regularly reveals significant information and concerns. This can provoke a complete re-evaluation of the assessment (it is similarly helpful at the end of follow-up appointments to ask 'Is there anything else you wanted to discuss?' Quite apart from ensuring thoroughness, such questions give an impression of unhurriedness).

Dr Coltrane feeds back his assessment to Mrs Mitchell, a full (rather than a capsule) summary. He is more or less obliged to give the patient a diagnosis, or at least a reframing of the problem as seen through his eyes. At this stage, the diagnosis or formulation is not always comprehensive or definitive. However, the patient wants to know what the doctor makes of her. It is a major agenda item. Such an explanation has to be both comprehensible and plausible to the patient. There is little point in telling someone with no psychiatric knowledge that they have a depressive illness without further explanation. It is more useful to explain that these particular symptoms are common, that they generally come as a group and that they are all part of depression. This is an illness insofar as it continues under its own momentum, even after the stresses that initially caused it have stopped. This is both in keeping with the psychiatric concept of the illness, and it is likely to make sense to Mrs Mitchell.

Main points in this chapter

1. Clinical interviewing is one of the main tools of the psychiatrist. Assessment interviews are daunting and strange to patients. They are more than an exercise in information gathering.
2. Patients and doctors enter clinical interviews with separate agendas. Each of them has preconceptions, which substantially affect the nature of the interview.
3. Both agendas are valid, but there is a tension between them. The main points in each agenda must be dealt with in the course of the interview.
4. Interviews move between different stages, which require different techniques.
5. Interviews are essentially interactive. Understanding the patient's experience of the interview assists the doctor in his task.
6. Assessment develops through hypothesis formation and testing.

Understanding and managing relationships with patients

Interactions between psychiatrists and their patients occur in the context of a therapeutic relationship. Sometimes the relationship is very brief. Sometimes the relationship lasts for many years. These relationships can go wrong. When they do, the problems usually have their origins in the beginning of the relationship, but only become evident far later.

All doctors have a responsibility to contain their relationship with their patient within distinct boundaries. This is a legal and ethical obligation. It is also crucial to the therapeutic effectiveness of the relationship. There are dilemmas in maintaining boundaries that cannot be resolved, but must be actively managed. On the one hand, the doctor must be concerned for, and interested in, the patient. He must be sufficiently giving of himself so that the patient feels able to trust him. On the other hand, the doctor must maintain a professional distance and bring a dispassionate objectivity to the relationship. He cannot let the patient enter his personal life. He must refrain from giving advice outside of his expertise. He must not let the patient's dependency grow to unmanageable proportions. Above all, he must not allow the therapeutic relationship to develop in such a way that it primarily serves his needs and not the patient's.

There are processes that operate within all therapeutic relationships that generate threats to the maintenance of boundaries. These threats include:

1. Transference reactions
2. Dependency
3. Identification
4. Breaches of confidentiality
5. The urge to rescue patients
6. Compromised truthfulness
7. Abuses of power

Each of these is considered below. There are also some dilemmas that commonly arise in clinical situations. These concern:

8. Gifts
9. Humour

10. Self-disclosure
11. Physical contact
12. Contact outside of the clinical setting
13. Termination

These are dealt with later in the chapter.

Transference reactions

Transference is a concept that was developed by Sigmund Freud. It has a particular meaning and importance in psychoanalysis. However, it is a common and observable phenomenon, which is important beyond the confines of specialist psychotherapy (Webster, 1995).

The patient usually has little information about the psychiatrist. The psychiatrist knows a lot about the patient, but the reverse is not true. The patient has no knowledge of the psychiatrist's personality and his life outside of his professional role. The psychiatrist is likely to play a significant role in the patient's life, at least in the short term. Understandably, the patient is driven to try and understand the psychiatrist as a person. The gaps tend to be filled by drawing on models set by significant people in the patient's past. For example, patients sometimes respond to the psychiatrist as if he is a judgemental and punitive parent, and react to quite neutral remarks with a defensive truculence. This draws on an example of middle-aged authority set by their parents. The doctor may have none of these parental characteristics, but in the absence of evidence, the patient behaves as if they have. This is transference as described by Freud. In practice, it includes other elements, for example, idealisation. All sorts of qualities can be attributed to the doctor in the absence of unambiguous evidence.

Dr Coltrane had a bad experience when he was 27 years old, three years through his psychiatric training. He was self-confident, and by now happy to work independently. He saw Mrs Chandler as a new outpatient. She was an attractive 34-year-old woman, with children aged 15 and 12. She had married young, and though her husband was a decent man, she had grown bored with him. When the children were small, he developed a domestic routine around the TV and the football, and he was content to carry on with this lifestyle now that the children were more independent. Mrs Chandler, on the other hand, was keen to have the active social life she missed when the children were young. She found a secretarial job, and flirting with the boss developed into an affair. She felt guilty about this, and she started to drink heavily. She became depressed, and eventually took a serious overdose whilst drunk.

Dr Coltrane saw her regularly in the clinic over the next few months. He helped her to stop drinking, and after some joint sessions with the couple, the marriage seemed to be improving. Mrs Chandler started to take more care over her appearance, which Dr Coltrane took to be a sign that she was less depressed. However, after an appointment when he told her that he felt she could be discharged, she confessed that she had resumed drinking. At the next appointment, she attended with her husband, who was surprised to hear about the drinking, as he had seen no evidence of it. A few weeks later, the drinking had reportedly stopped, but Mrs Chandler took a small and entirely unexpected overdose. Eventually, Dr Coltrane told her that he was leaving his post for a similar one at a nearby hospital. Mrs Chandler told him she did not want to see another psychiatrist, and they agreed that she should be discharged. She unexpectedly turned up at his final clinic and seemed flustered. She hastily handed him a letter and left. Dr Coltrane opened the letter at lunchtime, and was shocked by its content:

Dear Dr Coltrane
Thank you for being a good doctor to me and helping me out of my problems in the first few months that I was seeing you. I have been misleading you recently so that you would keep seeing me. The fact is I love you, and I think that you have some feelings for me. I have sat in your room longing to hold you. Doctors can't have relationships with patients, but I'm not your patient now. Please call this number. I'll be waiting to hear from you.
Love Tracey

Dr Coltrane took the letter to his consultant, Dr Davis, who was amused. The reception staff at the clinic had told him some weeks before that Mrs Chandler was besotted with Dr Coltrane. He had thought that Dr Coltrane was aware of this. On Dr Davis' advice, Dr Coltrane wrote her a very dry letter explaining that patients often develop strong feelings about their doctor. He pointed out that she knew very little about him, and bluntly stated that further contact between them would be inappropriate. He suggested that, if this distressed her, she should contact Dr Davis.

Dr Coltrane felt that he had made a huge mistake, and that this was bound to have an adverse effect on the patient. He also felt oddly violated, and was very uncomfortable at receiving an unwanted and taboo sexual advance.

The problem had its origins in the fact that Dr Coltrane had rendered himself oblivious to Mrs Chandler's behaviour towards him. At the beginning he felt that Mrs Chandler was attractive, and he dealt with this by ignoring it. In his efforts to respond to the patient in an entirely non-sexual and appropriate manner, he had driven her seductiveness from his awareness.

Mrs Chandler was not a sexual predator. Grateful to be feeling better, she had idealised Dr Coltrane. Although not especially good-looking, he seemed clever and kind. She imagined he had an exciting life, free of boring domesticity. Unable to read his responses to her, and in the absence of a clear message that Dr Coltrane was not sexually available to her, she escalated her signals to the point of explicitness.

The warning signs were obvious. If he had allowed himself to spot them, Dr Coltrane could have confronted her over-attachment. Given some time, it might have been possible to manage the relationship in a therapeutic way. On the other hand, if Mrs Chandler had known a little bit more about him, her fantasies might not have run so wildly out of control. This, however, would have had implications of its own for their relationship.

Dependency

Dependency is an inevitable development in a therapeutic relationship that the patient finds helpful, but it must be properly managed. It is the converse of transference, where strong feelings about the doctor are constructed largely from the patient's fantasies. Dependency occurs as the patient gets to know the psychiatrist as a person, and comes to feel that their well-being in the real world is contingent upon contact with him. Knowledge of the doctor as a person makes transference problems less likely, but it promotes dependency. The problem with dependency is that it undermines the patient's confidence in their ability to find their own solutions to problems, and it can be burdensome, and sometimes intrusive, for the doctor.

Mrs Redding is a 30-year-old married woman. Her husband is fifteen years older, and has grown-up children from a previous relationship. The couple is childless, a vasectomy reversal having failed. Mrs Redding has suffered panic attacks and episodes of low mood since her teens. She is close to her mother and sees her every day. She has always looked to her mother for advice. She is a very regular attender at her GP's surgery. One day, she consults her GP about an episode of palpitations. She has difficulty in accepting that the symptom is related to anxiety. Exasperated, the GP refers her to the local consultant psychiatrist, Dr Parker.

Dr Parker sees Mrs Redding in a busy outpatient clinic. The problem seems straightforward. Although the interview is relatively brief, he is satisfied that he has made a full assessment and established an appropriate treatment plan. He is aware that Mrs Redding is likely to remain anxious indefinitely, and he anticipates seeing her on only three or four occasions.

Although the consultation is somewhat hurried, Mrs Redding is very happy with it. She feels a good deal better immediately. Dr Parker seems to have grasped the heart of her unhappiness. She is sure he can help her. At the next appointment she reports improvement. Returning after a further month, things have deteriorated. Dr Parker explores recent events, and identifies a row with her stepdaughter as the cause of the problem. Mrs Redding finds this helpful, and feels better. A pattern in the treatment is established whereby Mrs Redding never improves for long enough for discharge. She is well satisfied with the treatment, as Dr Parker seems always to be able to understand what is bothering her.

Meanwhile, Dr Parker is happy to see Mrs Redding. She never wants much time, and she is always grateful for seeing him. He recognises that most exacerbations of symptoms are related to her inability to set limits on her stepdaughter, who abuses her hospitality and causes trouble between the couple. After unsuccessfully trying to get her to work out a strategy to deal with this, he increasingly gives direct advice on how Mr and Mrs Redding can together contain the stepdaughter's behaviour. By and large, his suggestions are effective, and the patient is so pleased that she brings other problems to Dr Parker for advice. Her husband starts deferring decisions until Dr Parker's views are known. Dr Parker is aware that Mrs Redding is dependent upon him, but a particular event makes him realise that he must do something about it.

A week after an appointment, Mr Redding phones him in his office. He tells Dr Parker that the couple really need his advice. The opportunity to move house has arisen, but they feel unable to make a final decision until they know Dr Parker's views. Will it have a good or bad effect on Mrs Redding? Naturally, Dr Parker does not know, but Mr Redding is a little put out when he declines to express an opinion.

Dr Parker is now forced to reflect properly on the state of this therapeutic relationship. He realises that Mrs Redding's anxiety symptoms are probably much as they have been for ten years. His personal involvement, far from being therapeutic, has burdened the couple with a dependency on him that has invaded their family life. It has undermined their ability to resolve difficulties and make decisions for themselves. Mrs Redding is perfectly happy with this, as it has made her feel more secure. It follows the familiar pattern of her relationship with her mother.

Dr Parker could allow things to drift on like this, but he feels that this would be irresponsible. At the next appointment, he explains to Mr and Mrs Redding what he feels has gone wrong. He makes a plan to discharge Mrs Redding after three further appointments. The couple are perturbed, but after two years of treatment, Mrs Redding is eventually discharged, reasonably happy, but with little change in symptoms.

Dr Parker is an experienced and skilled psychiatrist, but he made some errors. When he first saw her, he could have foreseen that Mrs Redding had a capacity to become very dependent. This was evident from the nature of her relationship with her mother. His first and biggest mistake occurred through haste. At the first interview, he had a clear plan for the duration of contact, but he did not clearly convey this. Within the therapeutic relationship, there was no clear treatment objective. Without this, Mrs Redding had an expectation that contact would be indefinite. For her, good relationships were characterised by dependency, and she had no way of knowing that this was inappropriate to the psychiatric setting. On the contrary, this was a particularly satisfactory dependent relationship, as Dr Parker brought an expertise and authority into her life that others lacked.

Dr Parker's second mistake was that, as he hurried through his clinics, he failed to notice that the relationship was drifting and purposeless. If he had stopped to review the situation after six months, he would have seen that he needed to take remedial action. As it was, he did not recognise this until the problem was severe.

Problems of this type are common, and they cannot always be neatly resolved. Many patients with long-term mental health problems, such as schizophrenia, must remain in follow-up indefinitely. Treatment involves mental health professionals directly in the patient's daily life. This means working within a dependency relationship. The dependency may be passed between different individuals occupying a single professional role, for example, community mental health nurse. These changes demand consistency with regard to the boundaries. Failures in boundary setting are more, rather than less, damaging in these situations.

Identification

It is not only patients who sometimes misconstrue therapeutic relationships. It is inevitable that psychiatrists will from time to time encounter patients with backgrounds similar to their own. The doctor and the patient may be struggling with similar problems in their personal lives. It is hard to avoid feeling a special kindred spirit with these patients. It sometimes seems that the patient's history casts a revealing light on the doctor's life. The mood of clinical interviews can subtly shift away from the professional towards something resembling a friendship.

There are considerable dangers in these situations. Firstly, hypothesising can break down. Identification leads to a loss of objectivity, and the psychiatrist starts making assumptions about the patient. The existence of parallels does not mean that everything is the same. Testing hypotheses is more important than usual, in order to avoid mistakes in assessment.

Secondly, the relationship is no longer truly patient centred, and an ambiguity can arise as to the purpose of the therapeutic relationship. This invites all the other types of boundary problems to occur. Even if this does not happen, the therapeutic nature of the relationship is compromised.

All psychiatrists will identify with some patients at some times. This need not lead to boundary breaches, provided that the psychiatrist has a degree of self-awareness. This issue is discussed at length in Part IV.

Breaches of confidentiality

In order to treat patients, doctors must be able to obtain sensitive personal information from them. Patients give the information on the understanding that confidentiality will be maintained. This protects the patient from the possibility that disclosures will leak out into the rest of their life, with adverse consequences.

Confidentiality is more complex than this reassuringly simple model. It is an active and dynamic issue between the doctor and the patient. Let us return to the interview between Dr Coltrane and Mrs Mitchell in the previous chapter. Mrs Mitchell was able to talk about herself knowing that doctors observe confidentiality. However, she had an implicit awareness that this confidentiality was not absolute. She was concerned that her children could be removed from her care as a consequence of her discussion with Dr Coltrane. In principle, she was correct. Where a doctor believes that a patient is seriously neglecting or abusing a child, he is obliged to override confidentiality and to take appropriate action to protect the child. This is a high-order legal and ethical obligation. Similarly, Mrs Mitchell was aware that psychiatrists can initiate admission to hospital under compulsion, another process that overrides confidentiality.

The awareness that confidentiality has limitations is widespread. It did not prevent Mrs Mitchell from being frank, but it did affect her agenda and the way that the interview proceeded. Patients do not imagine that confidentiality is absolute, and if they want absolute confidentiality, they will seek assurances prior to disclosures. Instead, there is an understanding that confidentiality is a high-ranking principle and that it will not be casually broken.

Confidentiality is attacked by many pressures external to the therapeutic relationship. Insurance companies, benefit agencies and others demand information that has been given in confidence. Patients permit the release of this information under duress, as otherwise they are denied their entitlements. Confidential information is shared between doctors and other health professionals, and is recorded in systems that are not 100% secure.

This emphasises the importance that individual doctors must attach to the maintenance of confidentiality at a personal level. Some psychiatric case histories make spectacular anecdotes. If such stories are related in a crowded restaurant, anyone overhearing is likely to lose faith in doctors' ability to be discreet. Within clinical teams, confidentiality issues must be constantly attended to.

Dr Parker sees a middle-aged woman with a history of childhood sex abuse and he describes this in his letter to the GP. The GP's receptionist reads the letter. When the patient next attends the surgery, the receptionist, in a quiet and kindly way, says 'Oh Eileen, you should have told us about that terrible business when you were a child'. The patient changes GP and never returns to the psychiatric clinic.

The urge to rescue the patient

Many people develop mental health problems in dreadful social or emotional circumstances. Mental illness not only causes them distress, it also restricts their ability to resolve their more tangible problems. Psychiatrists aim to relieve symptoms through psychological, social or pharmacological interventions. As the patient's mental state improves, they become able to act autonomously to resolve the problems in their life, which in turn reduces the stresses that exacerbate mental illness.

There is sometimes a temptation in the psychiatrist to move beyond their appropriate role, and to take on personal responsibility for rescuing the patient from their circumstances. This can take many forms. Interviewing a patient's parents and criticising them in the role of the patient's champion is not generally helpful; facilitating change within a family from a neutral position, by providing information or clarifying communication, is much more effective. There is an essential difference between ensuring that a patient claims his full welfare benefit entitlement and providing false information to a welfare agency, in order to help him to secure benefits beyond entitlement.

When one starts to feel the urge to rescue the patient, there is a prima facie case that the therapeutic relationship is going wrong. Boundaries will be breached unless the psychiatrist stops to consider what it is that is driving the urge.

Compromised truthfulness

The doctor's duty to be truthful guards a boundary both with individual patients and with society in general. At an individual level, doctors cannot help their patients if their truthfulness is in doubt, or if they protect patients from unpalatable truths. Society trusts doctors to be truthful. A medical report carries a gravity that is contingent upon its truthfulness being beyond doubt. It may occasionally seem that compromising one's truthfulness will help an individual patient, but once discovered, there is considerable damage to one's individual credibility, and to the credibility of the profession as a whole.

Mr Baker, suffering from anxiety, is referred to Dr Parker. He has witnessed a homicide, and he is frightened of the consequences of giving evidence. He requests a letter to the court to say that he is too unwell to give evidence. Dr Parker declines, because it is not true. Although it will be unpleasant and frightening for Mr Baker to give evidence, he is capable of doing so. Avoidance will only worsen his anxiety. If it were to become known that Dr Parker is willing to give untruthful letters of this sort, there would be a real risk of future witnesses being intimidated into seeing him to this end.

Abuses of power

Doctors wield power over their patients. They are well-educated, well-paid and they are afforded a range of privileges. Patients tend to trust them. A patient will allow a doctor to perform an intimate examination on first meeting and with minimal explanation. The patient cannot necessarily distinguish between a breast examination carried out for clinical reasons and one carried out for the doctor's sexual gratification. Nonetheless, many women will unquestioningly submit to the procedure. This combination of trust and power can be abused, sometimes with catastrophic consequences.

Dr Evans was a middle-aged psychiatrist with a drink problem. He spent his evenings drinking morosely in his study. At work, he isolated himself from his colleagues and stopped attending meetings. The part of his job that he really enjoyed was his Sexual Dysfunction Clinic. He felt he had special expertise, and was able to help ordinary couples in a way that made a real difference to their lives.

Some couples who attended his clinic could not readily grasp what was being asked of them. Sensate focusing was far removed from their concept of sex. To overcome this, Dr Evans would demonstrate for the couple. He would caress the woman's shoulders whilst pressing his chest against her back. On one occasion he lightly stroked the underside of a patient's breasts. Neither partner objected. He began to incorporate this into his treatment routine. He found this exciting, but he felt it was a legitimate procedure.

Eventually, he tried something similar when a patient complained that she could not introduce the smallest dilator for vaginismus. With her partner present, he demonstrated to them how the implement could be gently introduced. This, too, was incorporated into his routine treatment.

One afternoon he had a few drinks at lunchtime. In the clinic, a lady with vaginismus turned up without her partner. He proceeded with his routine as usual. Suddenly and impulsively, he dispensed with the dilator and used his fingers. The incident was quickly over and the patient seemed unperturbed. Dr Evans had become unequivocally sexually abusive, and there were more victims. He explained to the couples that he needed to do 'the gynaecological part of the treatment' with the woman alone. Many women submitted.

Eventually, there was a complaint and an investigation. Dr Evans lost his job and was struck from the medical register. He told his friends that he was the victim of a campaign of vilification. He may have been unwise, he said, but at the end of the day he had done nothing wrong.

This fictional story makes uncomfortable reading, and the circumstances are remote from the experience of contemporary psychiatrists in training. We include it because such occurrences are the worst possible outcome of a breach of professional boundaries. It involves an ordinary doctor, a man with problems, but not an intrinsically bad or evil man. Patients and their families can be irretrievably damaged in such circumstances.

These incidents really do happen, often to the amazement and horror of colleagues. Trainees, too, can run into trouble with the sexualisation of therapeutic relationships. The doctors involved rarely recognise the abuse of power involved, but it is invariable.

Two factors made Dr Evans especially dangerous. His isolation from his colleagues removed him from peer support and supervision. Everyone needs this. In its absence, he could ignore his first transgression of the boundaries, namely sexually touching a patient in a way that gave him pleasure. His capacity for *post-hoc* rationalisation allowed him to become a scheming sexual predator, whilst persuading himself and his patients that he was still acting as a caring professional.

Although other types of abuses of power are less dramatic (for example, financial dealings with patients), they frequently turn on similar dynamics and are always damaging to patients. Rationalisation of the abuse is particularly dangerous, as it is frequently the last of a series of breach of boundaries. It allows the doctor to serve his own needs at the cost of his patients.

Dilemmas in the maintenance of boundaries

There are a number of commonly occurring dilemmas, which highlight the difficult judgements that must be made in guarding the boundaries of the therapeutic relationship.

Gifts

Patients frequently offer psychiatrists gifts as a token of gratitude for their help. In other walks of life, this is unremarkable. For the psychiatrist, accepting a gift from a patient creates a real dilemma. Patients often offer a small and inexpensive gift at the end of a successful treatment. It has an importance for them as a social ritual, marking the end of a relationship that has resolved a problem for them. It creates a balance in a situation where there was a skew. The doctor has given something to them, and they have given something back. It allows them to part as a restored social equal. Refusal of such a gift causes offence and mars the termination of treatment.

Some patients offer gifts that are extravagant or excessively personal. Others give gifts regularly. Accepting these gifts is problematic. Mostly, patients give them because they like their doctor, but there may be other motives and other meanings. Some patients seek to create an indebtedness or special status for themselves, to be cashed in at a later time. Some patients are attempting to enter the doctor's personal life. Some insecure patients feel that gifts are needed to retain a relationship with the doctor. The gift symbolises a developing problem in the relationship.

In all cases, the doctor has to consider why this patient is offering a gift at this time. He must be prepared to discuss this with the patient. Inappropriate gifts should be refused, even if the patient is insistent. Most employers have policies forbidding the acceptance of any but the most trivial gifts, and the patient should be told this. Most importantly, one should never imagine that accepting a gift is of no significance. The doctor must always try to understand what it means.

Humour

Laughter and humour are important parts of discourse. They can defuse tensions, they can be used to vividly illustrate a point, and they can improve rapport within a relationship. Within teams they can improve morale and team spirit, and act as a foil to the grimness of some aspects of psychiatric work.

However, humour often has a hostile edge; someone is the butt of it. Laughter at what a patient has said may be offered warmly by the doctor, but may be taken as derisive or dismissive by the patient. Anxious and depressed patients may be unable to grasp the point of a joke, leaving both doctor and patient feeling awkward. A humorous remark reveals a lot about the teller's underlying values and beliefs, and once these are exposed, they may irreversibly change the relationship with the patient. The doctor's position of non-judgemental neutrality is important to the patient's willingness to expose their most private concerns, and once this position is lost, it cannot be recovered. Most humour has an element of ambiguity or wordplay, which psychotic or paranoid patients are likely to misinterpret. In teams, humour can run out of control, and teasing can proceed to bullying. An impression of flippancy can develop. Laughter and humour are powerful tools and must be treated with respect, as they can cause harm.

Self-disclosure

Patients grow curious about their psychiatrist, especially if they know them for a long time. They piece together facts learnt from other patients and from overheard conversations. It can be alarming to discover that a lot of information about you is in the public domain.

On meeting a new patient, he says that you have treated his aunt for years, that she says you are very nice, that he gathers you are married with two children and that you support Manchester City Football Club. He is a United fan himself. It later emerges that he knows that you are an atheist, whereas he is a Catholic. None of this is a disaster for the therapeutic relationship, but it does mean that you are not starting with a blank sheet. There are some potential issues that may arise later, for example, he may feel unable to comfortably discuss some worries he has about his social contacts at the church, feeling that you will not understand.

This process of prior knowledge is inevitable, and usually only becomes a major problem once you have a permanent post. However, trainees often become consultants in one of their training hospitals, and the leakage of personal information often starts during training. Consequently, it is as well to assume that anything you reveal about yourself will become part of accumulated folk knowledge. Your home address, revealed to one patient, might as well be given to all patients. The greater the patient's knowledge of you, the more difficult it is to maintain your position as a neutral figure.

Patients will often confront psychiatrists with a request for a personal disclosure: Are you married?, Are you a parent?, Are you a Christian?, Where are you from? This can mean that they feel you will not understand some part of their life unless you have the same beliefs or experiences as them. It is self-evident that you hardly ever meet a patient with identical beliefs and experiences as yourself. The psychiatrist's ability to understand his patient rests on factors other than similarities between them. Most psychiatrists are reluctant to make such disclosures, but try to explore with the patient why they have asked. This is a boundary issue, the message to the patient being 'In this setting, I put my personal beliefs to one side and I do not judge.'

Some psychiatrists feel that patients have a right to know some basic facts about them, and will make disclosures, but they still need to tackle the underlying issue in much the same way. Furthermore, they must carefully guard against advocacy of their political or religious beliefs, which is an abuse of power.

Finally, the doctor can offer self-disclosure as a means of powerfully illustrating a point. For example, Mrs Johnson is depressed and very troubled that she has developed checking rituals. Dr Coltrane says that this will resolve when she feels less depressed, but Mrs Johnson is not reassured. Dr Coltrane tells her that these symptoms are extremely common in the general population, and that he gets them himself when under stress. When he is very busy, he has to check the car doors and all the house locks before he can go to sleep.

However, it can easily go wrong. Mrs Johnson may feel that Dr Coltrane's symptoms are much milder than hers, and that he does not understand or that he is trivialising the problem. She may feel that the disclosure indicates that Dr Coltrane has problems, and that she should not burden him with her own. Dr Coltrane may have fallen victim to the trap of mistakenly identifying with the patient's problem. Mrs Johnson may actually have a range of undisclosed symptoms of chronic OCD. In leaping to this identification and disclosure, he has foreclosed further exploration of the symptoms.

Voluntary self-disclosure should be used sparingly and only where the doctor is certain that it is pertinent and appropriate to the patient's situation. It must not be used if the doctor himself is struggling with significant problems. This invites a collapse of the therapeutic relationship and even a reversal of care, where the patient feels responsible for the doctor's well-being. If in doubt, it is best not to do it at all. If one does make a disclosure, it is important to be vigilant for an alteration in the quality of the relationship.

Physical contact

People vary in their social use of touch. Within the dominant British culture, touch indicates intimacy. Outside of this, it is confined to stiff social rituals, such as shaking hands, or special situations such as goal scoring on the football field. Even small breaches of the no-touch rule cause significant awkwardness. A brief lingering of a handshake can feel very inappropriate to an Englishman. Other cultures, of course, follow entirely different rules. The degree of ordinary social touching prevalent in parts of the USA feels intrusive and socially promiscuous to a Briton.

This means that socially tactile doctors have to restrain themselves in clinical settings, as touch can create confused communications. The implication of intimacy may be experienced by the patient as invasive. It may draw the patient into an inappropriate familiarity or dependency. It may promote an abuse of power.

The appropriate use of touch is where the patient is distressed. A hand on the forearm can convey concern and can be comforting where verbal communication has, for the moment, become impossible. It must be unambiguous, which usually means that the patient is of the same sex or considerably older than the doctor. The contact should be brief. Protracted hand-holding is not generally therapeutically helpful. If one is uncertain if it will be well received, it is best not to touch.

Patients break the no-touch taboo when disinhibited. It is not a pleasant experience to be forcibly kissed by someone who is manic. As far as possible, such advances should be repelled, and you should make it clear that your personal space must be respected. This demands reciprocation; you have to respect your patient's personal space.

Contact outside of the clinical setting

It is inevitable that psychiatrists will occasionally meet patients and their families away from work. They may bump into each other in the street, or come across the patient in their own occupational role. Most patients will acknowledge the doctor as an acquaintance. Some wish to act as if they do not know the psychiatrist, and this must be respected as an aspect of confidentiality. Consequently, the doctor has to await the patient's social cue before either returning a greeting or doing nothing. Some patients are more effusive. They want to update the doctor on how they are doing, or they invite a change of relationship from therapeutic to social ('let's go for a drink!'). They may want to introduce the doctor to their friends. Mostly, such approaches are friendly and are not recognised by the patient as inappropriate. However, quite apart from the hazards for the therapeutic relationship, most of us do not want work to invade our own time. Fortunately, a courteous greeting and a determined moving on usually curtails the interaction and the patient is not offended.

Termination

Therapeutic relationships need a satisfactory conclusion. If they end abruptly, the patient can feel abandoned and rejected. Therapeutic progress can be lost. Abrupt termination of the relationship can arise in two ways. The first is where the doctor is leaving and neglects to inform the patient of this. Trainees move between posts, and they must give patients ample warning that they are going to leave. Inexperience leads trainees to underestimate their personal importance to their patients.

The second scenario arises when the therapeutic relationship has gone wrong, and the doctor withdraws in exasperation or panic. Unless there is a threat of actual violence to the doctor, abrupt termination is a self-indulgence that should be avoided. Even where withdrawal is the right outcome, as with Dr Parker and Mrs Redding, a little time is needed for the patient to understand and for the relationship to conclude.

A personal style

Understanding the main issues and pitfalls in managing therapeutic relationships helps the psychiatrist to find an appropriate personal clinical style. Some psychiatrists attempt to affect a dispassionate and distant clinical persona, following rigid and inflexible rules. Whilst this protects them from breaches of boundaries, it is rarely effective. The overall effect is cold and autistic, and it can cause considerable problems in establishing therapeutic relationships.

One brings one's own personality into the consulting room, with its strengths and its weaknesses. Effective clinical styles are built on this foundation. There is no single correct way of doing things, and no advice as to how to conduct oneself will work for everyone all the time. Any style will have some drawbacks. Opaque and reserved psychiatrists tend to encounter transference problems. Open and demonstrative psychiatrists tend to encounter dependency problems. It is important that psychiatrists should possess a high degree of self-understanding and maintain a critical awareness of what is going on within each therapeutic relationship. They must be ready to adjust their approach according to the nature of the patient's problem, and in the light of what happens over time.

Main points in this chapter

1. The rules of professional behaviour establish boundaries to therapeutic relationships that must be guarded by the doctor.
2. Guarding these boundaries creates dilemmas.

3. Breaches of boundaries tend to occur insidiously, and without vigilance they can go unnoticed. Even in the absence of professional misconduct, the consequence can be damaging to the patient.
4. When cases go wrong, review sometimes reveals an unwitting boundary breach. Recognition of this can guide remedial action.
5. Rationalisation of boundary breaches invites repetition and is a dangerous pattern.

Part III

The difficult interview

Not all interviews are easy to conduct. This section concerns the types of interviews which inexperienced interviewers find most anxiety provoking and troublesome. One way of understanding why these interviews are difficult is that there are hard-to-reconcile differences between the professional's and the patient's agendas. Once these differences are recognised, it may be possible to fully or partially resolve them. What is quite certain is that difficult interviews can only be successful when the interviewer has a clear understanding of the patient's likely motivations and points of view.

7

Difficulties relating to psychosis

A wide range of health professionals struggle to achieve satisfactory interviews with psychotic patients. If doctors in general are guilty of failing to see things from their patients' point of view, this is particularly true when the patient is psychotic. The term 'psychotic' is often taken to imply that the patient's viewpoint can be ignored. Psychotic patients are still sometimes treated by psychiatrists as if they are oblivious, only being addressed directly in order to demonstrate psychopathology.

Psychosis affects all aspects of mental functioning. However, personality does not disappear during episodes of psychosis. It is possible to make contact with the person despite the derangement. Events during psychosis are part of the person's life history and they have a significant impact after recovery.

This is not to deny that it can be very difficult to understand psychotic patients, though it is rarely impossible. However, one cannot expect to form useful relationships with floridly psychotic people if one lacks a basic understanding of what it is like to be psychotic.

The term 'psychosis' embraces a wide range of mental states. There are no general statements about it that do not have significant exceptions. Acute schizophrenia is a useful example of psychosis, as it is both common and difficult to understand. There are limitations in taking such an example. Not everything stated here holds true under all circumstances.

Acute schizophrenia involves more than a combination of delusions and hallucinations. It is a profound disorder of basic mental functioning. Psychiatrists believe that the problem is one of brain dysfunction. This view was once controversial, but it is now generally accepted that something goes seriously wrong with the fundamental operations of the cerebral hardware. However, psychosis occurs in the context of meaningful stresses and important situational problems. Psychotic ideas are often understandable in these terms. Although the mental state abnormalities are due to more than a psychological reaction, the things that psychotic patients say remain meaningful (Laing, 1990).

Psychiatric research into schizophrenia endeavours to identify sub-types, symptom clusters and underlying causes. The epidemiology of the disorder, and those factors that worsen or relieve the symptoms, are investigated. It is hoped that this knowledge will lead to more effective treatments and eventually to prevention strategies. Although such research is important, it casts little light on the subjective experience of being psychotic. Understanding the patient's experience is an important part of forming a therapeutic relationship with them.

Psychological understanding is based on observation and empathy, but it may be improved if one has access to an explanatory framework. The problem with such explanations is that they are speculative, and cannot be regarded as objective fact. They can only be tested against the criterion of utility. If one mistakes such explanations for scientific evidence, there is a danger of allowing a personal attachment to the theory to have the opposite effect to that intended; the relationship with the patient can be damaged, not improved. Box 7.1 summarises the ideas that we have found most useful in understanding our patients suffering from schizophrenia. Other clinicians have found a range of other frameworks helpful, and we make no claims for the superiority of ours.

The experience of being psychotic does not conform closely to popular concepts of madness. The man who thinks he is Napoleon and organises the Russian campaign from his garden shed is a stereotype that does not occur in real life. People do not become lost in coherent delusional worlds, they exist in the here and now, their usual personalities and habits moving in and out of focus as they struggle to cope with their mental dysfunction and the demands of reality.

People with chronic schizophrenia can be entirely normal in their demeanour, coping well with the nuisance of hallucinations, and holding delusional beliefs that are no more important than unusual opinions. In acute psychosis, the situation is different. The disorder is pervasive and yet fluctuating. The patient is aware of the real world and is capable of responding to it, but the capability is impaired and intermittent. Rudeness, disrespect or brutality have their usual effects on a psychotic person and are rarely forgotten or forgiven when psychosis passes.

A patient with acute schizophrenia

Gavin was 16 years old when his parents noticed that he was becoming quieter. He stopped playing football for the school team for no obvious reason. He started spending long periods in his bedroom listening to music. His school performance deteriorated, and his attendance became erratic. His parents felt that something was worrying him, perhaps his lack of a girlfriend, but even tactful questioning led to angry denials and periods of silent hostility.

BOX 7.1 Acute schizophrenia: a brief explanatory framework

The fundamental disorder at the heart of the schizophrenic experience seems to be 'psychotic turmoil'. It has its origins in a range of profound impairments, including disturbances of sensory filtering and interpretation. Thinking is disordered. It lacks goal direction and the logical syntax is impaired. Thoughts are connected in ways that are hard for others to understand. There is an inability to distinguish core and peripheral aspects of ideas. This causes problems in the evaluation of the outside world. Whilst associations between ideas become loose, concepts become more concrete. Emotions lose coherence and become disconnected from related thoughts.

The condition develops slowly, over many months. There is absolutely no reason why the sufferer should understand that the problem is with them rather than with the outside world. The changes are initially subtle, and there are no obvious florid symptoms, which arise much later. The person struggles to make sense of the world. Everything seems changed in an indefinable way, and this feels threatening. The subtleties of interaction become confusing. This creates a feeling that something critical or unpleasant is being said or implied by others beyond the actual words. Emotional arousal increases and this makes it still harder to function. To those around the person, he seems changeable. He often seems vague and distracted, at other times anxious or irritable for no clear reason. Sometimes he seems almost his normal self. It is hard for others to tell what is wrong.

Eventually, living with such a mental state becomes very frightening. In the absence of coherent thought or feelings, the person is unable to distinguish what is arising from within himself and what is arising externally. The sense of a continuous and whole self is threatened. The sense of self is a central part of mental functioning, a fundamental psychological construct that allows humans to learn and interact. Many of the florid symptoms of schizophrenia may be understood as an attempt to restore the core sense of self. The following are the key characteristics of the sense of self.

1. The sense of self is continuous. We carry a historical narrative that tells us what has happened in our life, what our enduring characteristics are, and how we come to be in this situation in the here and now. The sense of self allows us to understand who we are, and to learn from new experience. It allows us to understand that we have not ceased to exist whilst sleeping.

2. The sense of self has to distinguish between self and non-self. We can then tell if a sensation has arisen internally or externally and distinguish, for example, between a headache and being hit over the head with a hammer. This involves reality testing, a process of applying schemata to test the plausibility of our ideas. We look for clues as to the origins of sensory information and examine reactions to our behaviour. It is commonplace to think that one has heard one's name called. On seeing that there is no one nearby, there is a realisation that it has been imagined. This is reality testing.

3. The sense of self is unitary. The diverse states and feelings that we experience belong to one integrated person.

As psychotic turmoil worsens and the sense of self starts to break down, the person is confronted with the abyss of personal annihilation; falling forever and falling to pieces.

This breakdown of the sense of self corresponds to the clinical presentation of acute hebephrenic schizophrenia. There is marked thought disorder, rapidly changing emotions, grossly disorganised behaviour, an inability to interact appropriately, but no clear-cut or stable symptoms such as delusions or hallucinations. It is not the case that all patients with schizophrenia move through a hebephrenic phase, but it is suggested that the florid symptoms represent an attempt to avoid this state.

People suffering from acute schizophrenia restore their sense of self at a cost. It seems that, confronted with frightening and unintelligible experiences, they make an unconscious manoeuvre of abandoning reality testing. The unpleasant and frightening thoughts and emotions are arbitrarily attributed to the non-self. This restores a coherent sense of self, with those incoherent aspects of experience located in the outside world. Of course, the perceived non-self now contains parts that are internal to the person, but they are now experienced as hallucinations, passivity experiences, thought broadcasting and so on. The person feels whole. Although being paranoid is in itself frightening, persecution is a framework that can be dealt with more easily than complete personal dissolution.

This provides an explanation as to why psychotic beliefs are held with abnormal intensity and conviction. They serve an important function to prevent the person's sense of wholeness or integrity from falling apart. Attempts by a therapist to undermine these paranoid defences will in turn undermine the patient's sense of self, and their condition will deteriorate. Attempts to help the patient contain and control their paranoid experiences, without trying to abolish them, will make the manoeuvre more effective and less disruptive in everyday life. This corresponds to the unfavourable response of patients with schizophrenia to psychoanalytically based treatments compared to a much more favourable response to cognitive–behavioural techniques.

Gavin certainly did not feel too good. He found it hard to concentrate and often fell into the grips of a miserable sense of confusion. Unable to make sense of what was wrong, he searched for meaning in metaphysical ideas. He became interested in philosophy and psychology, and flicked through books for hours whilst alone in his room. Sometimes, a particular turn of phrase or a concept seemed to sum up what was wrong with the world, and he would feel briefly elated, but when he tried to explain his insights to others, the ideas would slip away from him and he was left with an empty feeling of puzzlement. Tasks, such as writing an essay, which once came easily to him, required tremendous effort. He felt uncomfortable around his friends, who seemed to be in on a joke which he could not understand. He felt most at ease when alone. It made him angry when people asked what was wrong. He did not know what was wrong, but it seemed to be related to the state of the world.

Eventually, his mother insisted on taking Gavin to their GP. She explained his change in behaviour. Gavin said he was fine, just a bit tired. The GP asked him about drug use, which he denied. On direct questioning, he confirmed that he was worried about not having a girlfriend and about his poor academic performance. The GP felt he was suffering from an adolescent stress reaction and he said to come back if things were no better in a few months.

Three months later, things were worse. Gavin had a continuous headache and a queasy sense of apprehension. Even minor decisions took a huge effort. He stopped attending school and he lay in bed trying not to think of anything. The rest of the house seemed alien and changed. He found it hard to understand what his parents were saying, and he felt sure that something awful was about to happen. He was dragged back to the GP, where he was sullen and miserable. The doctor felt that he was now frankly depressed, and prescribed an antidepressant.

Although Gavin protested that there was nothing wrong with him, his mother pressed him into taking the tablets. After a few days, he seemed to be improving. He started going out again. Three days after starting the tablets, Gavin noticed that an old Pink Floyd record contained a special message for him. It implied that he had a responsibility to prevent the destruction of the planet. At first he was relieved to find a meaning in all the confusing changes that had been going on around him. He started to notice more messages, and felt that he had to visit various places he had known as a child. People were looking at him oddly, and he felt that they could read his thoughts. A voice started giving him advice and instructions, sometimes friendly, sometimes threatening. Although he was frightened, life seemed meaningful and his terrible lethargy had lifted.

When Gavin's parents overheard him laughing to himself in his room, they started to feel really worried. Now when they questioned him, he angrily insisted that they knew perfectly well what was happening. One evening, he stormed into the house and demanded that his parents give him the 'heart key'. He became frustrated at their inability to understand and he threw a clock through a window.

The following day, Gavin was lying on his bed, listening to his radio. He had tuned between stations and was listening to a voice that he could hear within the white noise, telling him that he would die sexually if he did not get the heart key. There was a knock at the door, and his mother walked in, followed by the GP and Dr Coltrane who was introduced as 'a specialist who has come to see you'. Gavin was angered by the sudden intrusion, especially as he needed to concentrate on the radio. He irritably ordered the threesome out of his room. He complained of their rudeness at coming uninvited and without a prior appointment. He turned the radio up and the voice warned him not to talk to the doctors who were trying to keep him away from the heart key.

Gavin was agitated by the turn of events. He felt torn between co-operation and withdrawal. He respected doctors, and he wanted to talk about what was happening to him. However, he did not know who Dr Coltrane was, and it was possible that he was a mind reader. The excitement of the moment set off a riot of fragmented thoughts and feelings. He had a strong urge to get out, if not through the door, then out of the window. He would like to sit down and explain, but just now he needed the chance to calm down. Dr Coltrane asked the others to leave and said that he would leave too, if Gavin insisted, but that it might be useful to talk.

The psychiatrist's agenda

Interviewing an acutely psychotic patient for the first time is different from an ordinary interview. Attempts to rigidly adhere to a standard format are doomed to failure. This is not to say that the systematic acquisition of information can be neglected. On the contrary, it is important to ensure that history is comprehensive, as it is likely to be delivered in a muddled way. Information is likely to come from a range of sources. Sometimes it takes several interviews to clarify important background history. The patient may not have come willingly. The doctor is likely to have significant information prior to speaking to the patient.

1. When interviewing someone with acute psychosis, the psychiatrist's agenda is dominated by the need to do something. The dominance of this item represents a major problem in establishing a therapeutic relationship with the patient. It is likely that the doctor will be prepared to force action on the patient if it proves impossible to reach a safe and satisfactory plan by agreement. The psychiatrist wants to contain the risk that the patient will harm himself or somebody else. In any case, he is likely to feel that the patient will only deteriorate without treatment. Family, friends or police are often involved and they are likely to press hard for some form of intervention. This agenda item dominates as soon as it is clear that the patient is psychotic, and long before assessment is complete. It can be reframed as the question 'What is an appropriate intervention, and how am I going to get the patient to accept it?'

2. The psychiatrist needs to understand the overall situation. He requires sufficient background information to understand who the patient is, what effect his illness has on his daily functioning and on those around him, what supports exist for him, and what concerns are held by those closest to him. Evidence of aggressive or self-harming behaviour is important, as is evidence

of self-neglect. Substance misuse is important, as it can lead to sudden alterations in behaviour, and can compound impaired judgement.

3. The psychiatrist wants to understand the patient's current mental state. This does not just mean eliciting psychopathology, but also understanding the patient's concerns and wishes. Understanding that a psychotic patient is concerned for the welfare of their cat, and that they will only go into hospital if the cat is properly cared for, can be an important component in achieving treatment on a cooperative basis. Psychopathology does matter. For example, command hallucinations or jealous delusions are associated with dangerous behaviour. However, there is much more to the psychotic patient than the sum of their symptoms.

4. An impression must be formed of the trajectory that the situation is following. This is not a term that is familiar from psychiatric textbooks, but it is a concept that is important to all practising psychiatrists. Trajectory includes both direction and speed. By taking all the available information together, it is possible to form an impression of how rapidly the situation is developing and whether adverse events are likely to occur. Both illness characteristics and contextual factors, such as the capacity of those coping with the situation to carry on in this role, are drawn together to assess trajectory. It is a key factor in deciding, for example, between inpatient and community treatment.

5. The psychiatrist is trying to win the patient's trust. He must not do this through trickery or dishonesty. It can be impossible to win a psychotic patient's trust. Where it can be achieved, it makes a substantial difference to the ease with which treatment proceeds and to the patient's experience of treatment.

6. If this fails, the psychiatrist wishes to have some authority in the situation. This does not correspond to being authoritarian, which tends to evoke hostility. It is helpful for the psychiatrist to be in charge in these situations in a way that would otherwise be quite inappropriate.

7. The psychiatrist wishes to conduct himself in a way that will withstand retrospective scrutiny. A therapeutic relationship cannot be built on foundations of patronising, dismissive or bullying behaviour. The doctor is at the start of a lengthy relationship with the patient. He must be able to justify to the patient what he has done and the manner in which he did it.

The psychotic patient's agenda

One cannot assume that this will be incoherent. The following is a list of agenda items that patients may bring to interviews. It is not exhaustive, and an individual will not carry them all.

1. Many psychotic patients engage in an interview with a psychiatrist because they have been told to do so. They follow a pattern of deference and social convention. They have no clear idea of the purpose of the interview, and they have no positive expectations of the outcome. This is anxiety provoking. Anyone would be anxious about an interview that has been arranged by someone else and without an evident purpose.

2. Many psychotic patients want something from the psychiatrist that is compatible with his agenda. They may simply want to unburden themselves, to talk with someone outside of the situation about the bad things that have been happening. They may want help with the situation. They are unlikely to see this in the same terms as the psychiatrist, but nonetheless, they may feel that he is an appropriate person to turn to for assistance. For example, paranoid patients may seek sanctuary through hospital admission in order to escape persecutors, rather than because they feel that they are ill. They may feel depressed and suicidal and want psychiatric help with this, rather than with the psychotic symptoms that are causing them to despair.

3. Psychotic patients sometimes want something from the psychiatrist that is not compatible with his agenda. For example, patients often want the psychiatrist to support their point of view, to agree that they are not unwell when others are suggesting that they are, or to confirm that their delusional beliefs are based on reality. They can demand inappropriate interventions, such as surgery to remove a radio from their abdomen or hypnosis to reveal a hidden truth.

4. Most patients are looking for someone they can trust, because they are frightened and confused and do not know what to do. It is hard to trust anyone when you are psychotic, but doctors have an advantage in winning trust because of the special status of the medical profession.

5. Believing that there is nothing wrong with them, some patients simply want to escape the psychiatrist's attention, to get out of the interview and to be left alone. This may take the form of wanting to explain that they are fine, but it may be much more hostile than this. Young men, wary of the police in general, and now taken against their will to hospital in a police van, are likely to view the psychiatrist as an arm of oppressive authority, and attempt to deal with him by silence or threats.

Reconciling the agendas

It may be impossible to completely resolve the conflicts between the psychiatrist's and patient's agendas in these situations. It is usually possible to reconcile enough to establish a therapeutically useful relationship, or at least to allow such a relationship to flourish at a later time. A permanent skew can enter into the relationship, with the patient permanently viewing the psychiatrist as a benign but controlling authority figure. Sometimes the relationship contains an element of permanent active hostility, though the expression of this varies over time.

There are two elements that assist reconciliation of agendas. One is the way that the psychiatrist conducts the interview, and the other is the active process of negotiation.

Conducting the interview

Successful interviews with psychotic patients do not require complex techniques. The main requirement is for a heightened attention to the ordinary rules of interviewing with some accommodation to the vulnerabilities and difficulties of someone who is acutely psychotic.

Psychotic patients cope badly with stimulating environments. They have particular problems with ambiguity and with distracting stimuli. Calmness and openness are helpful. Familiar social behaviour is reassuring, whilst anything suggestive of covert motives or frank trickery is alarming.

There is a need to consider the setting in which one conducts the interview. The doctor often finds himself in an environment over which he has little control, such as an Accident and Emergency (A&E) Department, the patient's home or a police station. Nonetheless, it is usually possible to take some steps to make the situation easier for the patient.

As far as possible, the interview should be conducted one-to-one and in privacy. This often means removing other people from the room. If the patient feels safer with a friend or family member present, this can be helpful, provided they are asked not to intervene (complex three-way dialogues are difficult for both the patient and the doctor). Interruptions from outside and extraneous noise are very unhelpful, and others should be asked to avoid this.

If the doctor is fearful, the patients will pick this up and become more fearful themselves. It is essential that the doctor feels safe. The interview should be unhurried, and the doctor should be firm but polite. Most patients who are psychotic are reassured by the feeling that the doctor is in control of the interview. The doctor should be as open as possible, explaining why he is there and what his concerns are. It must be clear that the doctor is listening sympathetically, neither challenging nor confirming delusional ideas. He must acknowledge the patient's distress and attend to the patient's realistic concerns. The doctor is looking for common ground during the interview, identifying those items in the patient's agenda which correspond to his own, in order to allow a negotiation.

Negotiating with psychotic patients

Negotiation implies that full reconciliation of agendas is not possible. In a negotiation, some agenda items have to be abandoned by one side or the other in order to achieve a plan of action that is acceptable to both parties. If this cannot be achieved, cooperation, which is normally a pre-requisite of doctor–patient relationships, will break down, temporarily or permanently. In practice either party can implement this; in the patient's case by running away, and in the doctor's case by initiating compulsory action under mental health legislation.

It is conventional to state that psychotic patients can be treated without compulsion, provided they have 'good insight'. Insight is, however, a difficult concept, hard to define and not located solely in the patient. Insight really means the degree to which the patient agrees with the doctor. 'Good insight' is the outcome of a negotiation between the doctor and the patient, aimed at finding an agreement as to what is wrong in order to work together. Insight is not a quality of the patient, but of the relationship.

The process of finding common ground is a dynamic one, with both doctor and patient playing an active role. Most patients feel that they have a problem, even if they believe it is external to them. There is little point in the doctor forcing a formulation of the problem that is totally unacceptable to the patient ('Well, actually it isn't the freemasons that are the problem. You have acute paranoid schizophrenia and you need hospitalisation'), but is also unhelpful to dishonestly collude with delusions ('The freemasons won't be able to get you on Ward 5'). The doctor must find a position that is honest but not confrontative. For example, 'You will feel safer on Ward 5'. This bypasses the question of belief in the delusion and establishes a truthful common concern. It implies that a problem is located in the patient, laying the ground for later negotiations.

Negotiations are necessary on all kinds of issues in the continuing relationship between the doctor and the patient, and often stretch far into the future. The principles are unchanging. The most serious pitfall is dishonesty. For example, it is very tempting to suggest that a patient should come into the hospital for a few days for a rest, in the hope that this sounds so innocuous that the patient will accept it. The doctor knows that the admission is likely to last weeks and that any attempt to leave will lead to detention. The 'few days rest' offer is unethical and causes problems later. When the patient finds he is unable to leave hospital, he is unlikely to easily trust the psychiatrist again. The admitting doctor has pulled an expedient trick on the patient that has persistent adverse consequences. Promises of rapid recovery, side-effect-free medication, or any other untenable undertaking will similarly damage long-term therapeutic relationships.

Detained patients

The detention of patients in the hospital is an unavoidable reality of psychiatric practice. Without detention, significant numbers of seriously ill patients would suffer, deteriorate or die. That small minority of psychotic patients, who are dangerous when unwell, would commit offences and be imprisoned.

Most psychiatrists dislike detaining patients. They recognise that once a patient has been detained, the therapeutic relationship is forever altered, though not necessarily destroyed. The knowledge that psychiatrists have the power to detain affects relationships with patients far beyond those who actually experience detention. Treating a patient under compulsion introduces a new agenda item into the relationship between the doctor and the patient, namely the issue of control.

The psychiatrist's power over detained patients is very extensive. Detention is a major event in the patient's life. However, it is a routine aspect of the psychiatrist's work. The psychiatrist is familiar with the psychiatric ward and becomes desensitised to the disturbed and disturbing aspects of this environment. Modern inpatient units are more attentive to patient's needs than mental hospitals were in the past, when patients had no rights and little ability to make complaints. Consequently, professionals tend to see detention as relatively benign, and lose sight of the nightmarish quality of the experience.

We usually think of freedom as a political issue, the right to free expression and free association. We tend not to think of more banal freedoms, which are only usually lost in the context of imprisonment. Detained patients, it can be argued, have less freedom even than a prisoner, and are held under far more ambiguous rules. The experience of being detained, coming together as it does with acute mental illness, is very frightening. The doctor may not feel powerful, but he is exerting extensive control over his patient. It is inevitable that the effect on the subsequent relationship is profound.

The experience of being detained

Gavin was admitted from home under compulsion a few days after the psychiatrist's visit. He had initially agreed to take medication, but never did. He had come to believe that his parents were mind-readers. In an argument, he threw a cup at his father, cutting his head. That evening he was arguing with the voice in the radio, which was telling him that he was about to die sexually, when there was some noise outside the house. He went out to find his parents, the doctors, two social workers, two ambulance men and three policemen in earnest discussion. Panic stricken, he rushed to his room. There was a series of shouted conversations through the locked door, with implausible reassurances followed by escalating threats of forced entry. A hastily constructed barricade of furniture proved inadequate when the police forced the door open. He was bundled down the stairs and into the ambulance in handcuffs, while he was screaming for help and pleading to be left alone.

The ward was institutional, despite homely touches and domestic furniture. The staff were calm and pleasant, but to Gavin it was obvious that they were part of the plot against him. He was extremely wary of them. He slept badly in a small dormitory full of strangers. Over the next few days, Gavin felt that his plight had worsened. He did not trust the staff, and the other patients were obviously mentally disturbed. He was told that if he tried to leave, he would be stopped, by force if necessary. There seemed little point in appealing for release to the same authorities that had acted against him. He was not allowed to collect his belongings from home, or to go to the local shops. He was forced to follow a routine of meal times that were rigid and against his normal pattern. He was not allowed to lie on his bed when he wanted to. He was allowed no privacy and was constantly observed by staff, even when washing. He was given tablets which he was told would make him feel better, but they made him drowsy. His hands shook and he felt constantly restless. His mouth was dry, but he could only have a cup of tea at certain times. He observed that refusal of tablets could lead to quite brutal forced injections. He had no idea why he was being held in these conditions. There was no indication as to what he had to do in order to be released, other than to submit to the regime. He soon abandoned protest and did as he was told. The situation was quite hopeless. His spirit was broken.

Compulsory treatment was the right thing in the circumstances, but it was still oppressive. No matter how humane the regime, it is inevitable that many patients find the experience similarly unpleasant. Gavin eventually recovered and told the psychiatrist that hospital admission had been the right intervention, but the impact of this exercise of power over Gavin remained within their relationship.

Long after release from hospital, the patient is aware that defiance of the psychiatrist's advice may lead to further detention. For the relationship to be helpful to the patient, this issue needs to be an open one. The doctor must make it clear from the outset why he thinks that detention is appropriate, what he thinks is wrong and the purpose and nature of the treatment. These have to be explained in terms that the patient can understand, which will vary over time. Even if the patient disagrees with what has been done, it is possible to have a therapeutic relationship on the basis that the doctor is well intentioned. The exercise of control is damaging when it appears arbitrary and capricious.

Some patients are reassured by being detained. When everything is frightening and out of control, it can be reassuring to return to a more child-like position where someone else takes charge and makes difficult decisions for you. Repeatedly detained patients can become quite dependent upon their psychiatrist, and one has to work within this dependency. It is not the same as the emotional dependency of the anxious outpatient, who needs to attend the clinic regularly in order to feel secure. For these more severely ill patients, the psychiatrist has a major impact on their material circumstances, not just in detaining them, but in helping them secure benefits, housing and daytime activities. They sometimes invite a doctor who has held them unwillingly in hospital to attend major life ceremonies, such as weddings and christenings.

Dealing with psychotic patients who are frightening

Most inexperienced doctors are uneasy when interviewing psychotic patients, but open fearfulness is unhelpful. Fear militates against careful listening and decision-making. A fearful doctor will make the patient feel worse. Fear raises the degree of emotional arousal in the interview. It creates ambiguities and a sense of insecurity that feeds patients' paranoid feelings.

Psychotic patients can be frightening even when they do not pose a threat to the doctor. The more a patient is similar to one's self, the less likely they are to invoke fear. Conversely, those types of persons who are most likely to cause apprehension in ordinary life seem most frightening when mentally disturbed. Differences in ethnicity and class can contribute to a fearfulness that is not necessarily related to any immediate realistic threat. One needs to be aware that fear may be more related to prejudice than to objective risk.

Unpredictability is frightening. Experienced psychiatrists are more comfortable than trainees in the presence of psychotic patients. Psychotic patients' behaviour is more predictable to doctors with a good understanding of psychotic mental states. Psychotic patients interact differently from other people. Their emotional rapport and body language are wrong, and this creates unease. They may be difficult to converse with. Their suspiciousness or perplexity is uncomfortable. Above all, states of over-arousal are intensely unsettling for the doctor. The patient is restless, tense, sweaty, and hypervigilant; the condition signals danger.

Psychotic patients can be aggressive or violent. In general, psychotic patients become aggressive because they are either frightened or because they are frustrated. The major exception to this are manic patients who in a state of elation and excitement may become indiscriminately aggressive as an intrinsic part of the mood abnormality.

Needless to say, the process of psychiatric assessment offers ample opportunity for a psychotic patient to become frightened or frustrated. Most patients who are going to be aggressive show clear signs of this by the time the psychiatrist arrives. One is often confronted by a very angry person at the beginning of the interview. It is unusual for aggression to arise afresh in the course of an interview.

The key to calming such patients is to be calm yourself. To achieve this, you must ensure that the degree of personal danger is minimal. You should refuse to conduct the interview until this is achieved. This insistence can create an uncomfortable impression of cowardice, especially within the macho culture of hospital medicine. It may mean refusing to see a patient who is at risk at home until others are available to attend with you. Failure to achieve this does the patient a disservice. The psychiatrist's interview and assessment are likely to have major consequences. They cannot be appropriately carried out by a doctor who is desperate to get away from the patient. The issue of safety is discussed in greater depth in Chapter 16.

Main points in this chapter

1. Interviews with patients suffering from acute psychosis require a different technique to other clinical interviews. The basic principles of the interaction and relationship are otherwise unchanged.
2. Psychosis can be understood. The patient's individual wishes and concerns remain meaningful, despite the mental state abnormality.
3. Psychiatric intervention may curtail the patient's freedom and autonomy. This damages the therapeutic relationship. The damage is minimised by retaining an awareness of how one's actions are received, and by engaging in a process of honest negotiation.
4. Psychotic patients can be frightening irrespective of the realistic danger. Measures that secure the doctor's safety facilitate a successful interview and serve the patient's best interests.
5. A mark of truly expert psychiatrists is their ability to converse with psychotic patients in a relaxed and normal way. To achieve this one needs a good comprehension of the subjective experiences of one's patients.
6. These interviews are difficult for doctors but they are considerably more difficult for patients.

8

Unpopular patients

Every psychiatrist could provide a personal list of types of patients they find problematic to treat. Such a list would be largely idiosyncratic and based on the psychiatrist's personality. Some psychiatrists like treating patients with eating disorders; others find such patients difficult and frustrating. Some find alcoholics self-indulgent and irritating whilst others enjoy treating them, and so on. This reflects variations of interest and aptitude which are natural. The positive aspect of this is that it leads to special expertise in treating specific disorders. This chapter is not concerned with these preferences. Some types of patients, on the other hand, have problems that create difficulties for most psychiatrists, in that it is difficult to form a useful therapeutic relationship with them. These individuals are sometimes called 'heart sink patients'. The terminology is revealing, as it implies that the difficulty is at least in part related to the doctor's emotional response. 'Heart sink' implies that they induce a sense of helplessness and frustration.

Dysfunctional doctor–patient interactions are characterised by a failure to find an accommodation between the doctor's and the patient's agendas. These patients often carry agenda items that they cannot or will not make explicit, but which are implicit in their behaviour. They cannot always be helped. An understanding of the dysfunctional therapeutic dynamic at least eases the doctor's sense of despair.

As in many dysfunctional situations in life, both parties in these unhappy clinical situations repetitively attempt to deploy strategies that have already failed. The trick is to find new, more adaptive strategies. Sometimes, the process of thinking about the problem differently will reveal a way forward to a more helpful interaction.

'Somatisers'

This commonly used term does not precisely correspond to 'those patients suffering from somatisation disorder'. 'Somatiser' is informal jargon. It refers to people who experience emotional distress as physical symptoms, or believe that their problem is wholly or in part due to physical disease, when the doctor believes it is psychological in origin.

The patient commonly arrives at the psychiatrist's office determined to prove that the condition is organic. They attend in angry submission to another doctor's insistence that they should have a psychiatric assessment. The patient may be worried that physical illness is going untreated. Even before the patient is seen the psychiatrist anticipates trying to persuade the patient that he is wrong. The doctor and the patient have agenda items diametrically opposed to each other. It is hardly surprising that such interviews are uncomfortable and frequently unproductive.

The behaviour of somatising patients suggests that they believe that physical distress is more authentic than emotional distress. They seem to feel that they can only be cared for if they are physically unwell. This is a *meta-agenda* that determines other specific agenda items, such as the search for an organic diagnosis. It is covert, hidden from the explicit content of the interview, and outside of the patient's immediate awareness. Such beliefs are sometimes culturally determined, and only cause problems where the doctor is from a different culture. Sometimes these beliefs have arisen developmentally in response to early emotional experience. In either case, such deep-seated attitudes are unlikely to change just because a psychiatrist says they are wrong. On the contrary, it is trying to persuade the patient that they are wrong that feeds and sustains the relationship, and keeps it dysfunctional.

In assessing 'somatisers', it is best to adopt a position of neutrality with respect to the nature of their problem. This can be made explicit at the outset with a statement to the effect 'I don't know what's wrong with you. Tell me the story from your point of view.' Without this, the doctor and the patient rapidly become locked in conflict. Unless there is a statement to the contrary at the outset, the patient will assume that the doctor has an opposite view to them, and act out their side of the conflict.

Clinical scepticism is a quality that protects psychiatrists against making mistakes. It is an attitude that insists on evidence and acknowledges uncertainty. It demands that you critically evaluate everything you are told, not in a spirit of cynicism, but in the recognition that human beings get things wrong. This includes health professionals. In treating somatisers, clinical scepticism demands a neutral position, because sometimes the patient is right. Doctors have a marked tendency to think that a problem is psychological if investigations prove negative. The diagnosis 'psychological problem' is a residual category, that which is left when other possibilities have been excluded. The psychiatrist, however, is looking for positive evidence, a plausible psychological formulation of the problem. In the absence of this, the problem may well be organic. In the fullness of time, an underlying organic problem sometimes becomes evident. A proportion of patients sent to psychiatrists with vague and allegedly psychogenic neurological symptoms turn out to have multiple sclerosis.

Many somatising patients have a combination of organic and functional problems. Patients with chronic low back pain often become very miserable because of pain and disability. There is no demonstrable back pathology and they are obviously depressed. It is often implied or frankly stated that there is nothing wrong with their back and that the problem is psychological. Not surprisingly, the implication that the problem is imaginary tends to make them angry and despairing. It seems unlikely that pain can be conjured in the total absence of a painful sensory stimulus. It is perfectly possible to sustain a soft-tissue back injury leading to muscle spasm, which hurts a lot. Soft-tissue injuries and muscle spasm do not show on X-rays. Efforts to avoid muscle spasm create postural stresses leading to further soft tissue damage and more muscle spasm. Depression and anxiety lead to a lowering of pain threshold.

The psychiatrist's neutrality over organicity can allow some patients to accept this type of mixed physical and psychological explanation, which then allows a useful therapeutic relationship to develop. However, there is not always such a plausible explanation available, and some patients are too entrenched in their conflict with the medical profession to concede even this degree of psychological causation. The psychiatrist's neutrality can allow a reframing of the problem under these circumstances. For example:

I can't do anything about your symptoms, because I don't understand what's causing them, but if you felt less tense about it all, you'd probably cope with the symptoms better.

These physical symptoms are outside of my expertise, but the problems between you and the doctors aren't helping at all. Maybe we can do something about that.

This type of approach works with a significant proportion of somatisers. There are treatment strategies that are effective, but they are beyond the scope of this book. In order to deploy them, one must form a cooperative relationship with the patient.

Patients who will not acknowledge that they have recovered

This is a problem that arises late in the therapeutic relationship. The doctor thinks the patient is better, but the patient will not agree. The problem can arise in a number of different ways and for a number of different reasons:

- Dependency difficulties, as in the case of Mrs Redding, described in Chapter 6. Some of these patients will state that they are well, but that they are fearful of relapse. They want continued contact in order to feel secure. The conflict in agendas here is that the doctor feels they have fully recovered, whilst the patient feels damaged by having been unwell. For them, the loss of symptoms does not equate with recovery.

- Seeking perfection: Some patients present new problems every time discharge seems imminent. A proportion of patients in the 'well but dependent' group will resist discharge in this way, but there can be different factors at play. Some patients have not shared the objective of simple symptom resolution from the beginning. They are seeking a more thorough improvement in themselves, an unrealistic hope of becoming more content with life and free of problems.

- Covert motivations for continued attendance: These include support for higher rates of benefit, rehousing, early retirement on medical grounds or the avoidance of punishment by the criminal justice system.

These problems turn on a single theme. The doctor and the patient have different objectives for treatment. The seekers of perfection have unrealistic expectations. The patients who find that the fact of psychiatric attendance resolves non-psychiatric problems are using the relationship inappropriately from the doctor's point of view, though not from theirs. It is hardly surprising that people struggling to survive on the margins of society will exploit any advantage they can find.

As with somatisers, there can be a meta-agenda behind the more obvious conflict. These patients bring to the interaction a model of doctor–patient relationship that is radically different to the psychiatrist's. For example, the role of carer is, for the doctor, a temporary state, with an objective (recovery) that creates a limit to the relationship. For some patients, however, being in a cared-for relationship is an end in itself. The relationship meets needs that are not otherwise satisfied. The therapeutic relationship does not facilitate change; it only solves a problem in the here and now, and therefore there is an expectation that it should continue. In contrast to this, some patients have such a low expectation of being helped by professionals that they see the doctor as someone who must necessarily be manipulated if they are to get anything worthwhile from the relationship.

Clarity at the outset with regard to the expected length and outcome of treatment helps to avoid this kind of difficulty, but the psychiatrist is still faced with some patients who have to be discharged more or less unwillingly. The trauma of forced discharge is eased if it is possible to identify, with the patient, the nature of the problem.

Patients who lie

Truthfulness is an elusive quality, which has more to do with intention than veracity. Very few of us are capable of complete openness even momentarily, and certainly not all the time. It is the intention to mislead that sets lying apart. Psychiatrists must be attentive to the possibility of lying. The attitude of unconditional positive regard, which is a tool of the trade, can make psychiatrists appear gullible. This is certainly preferable to the appearance of being a doubting inquisitor. It is clinical scepticism that protects psychiatrists from being misled. Clinical scepticism demands answers to questions such as: Does this story make sense?, Do the dates of events leave major gaps unaccounted for? and Is the patient's account consistent with other accounts? These questions can raise the possibility that the patient is lying.

Psychiatrists cannot allow themselves to be outraged by lying. The untruthfulness may not be deliberate. It may arise because the truth involves a sensitive secret. The process of teasing out the reasons for the untruth, and the significance of the truth, are grist to the mill in helping the patient. There is a large group of patients who complain of hearing voices without displaying other psychotic symptoms. It is often said that they are 'putting it on'. Not everyone who hears voices is psychotic, and it is wrong to assume that they are lying. Within this group, there are some individuals who go on to develop schizophrenia.

Patients who deliberately and determinedly lie carry a meta-agenda, which is similar to that carried by patients who wish to stay in follow-up for manipulative ends. They feel impotent. They do not believe that they will be accepted or helped if they reveal themselves as they really are. They fear that they will be rejected, or believe that they must manipulate and control other people in order to get anything from them.

Confronting patients when you are sure or almost sure that they are lying is not easy, as open disbelief compromises the doctor's neutrality and unconditional positive regard. Blunt confrontation will lead the patient to withdraw from treatment, or to the replacement of the first lie with a second lie. Untruths can be disentangled without a direct accusation. Puzzlement at inconsistencies (the 'Colombo' posture), and a refusal to be deflected from understanding these, will often eventually lead to the truth. Sometimes, the patient is so resistant that there is no alternative to stating that you feel that they are not being entirely truthful. This cannot be executed as a hostile confrontation. A constructive confrontation requires a much more neutral form of interaction, despite its intrinsically accusatory content. This takes a little practice to get right.

Some patients tell really big lies. Sometimes these are easily detected. False accounts tend to be dramatic and therefore implausible ('my whole family died in

an air crash last week') or inconsistent with the verifiable facts. Full-time malin-
gerers, for example patients with Munchausen syndrome, are few in number,
but they get around a lot, and psychiatrists deal with them quite commonly.
A few of them become very accomplished at their art, and there is little that the
psychiatrist can do to avoid being misled by them. These pathological liars are
almost impossible to work with. They usually flee on being caught out, but some
just invent another elaborate story.

Patients who persistently complain

These days, complaints against doctors and medical services are encouraged, and
rightly so. The failings of professionals can have a serious impact upon their
patients. However, there is a small group of patients who are habitual users
of complaints systems. Their persistent complaints about their treatment can
reflect a problem with them, rather than with the professional.

These patients are often referred after they have fallen out with their previous
psychiatrist. They ask for a change of doctor, or the previous psychiatrist has
had enough and has discharged them. Although they may express doubt as to
your usefulness at first meeting, they more often state an expectation that you
will prove more satisfactory than the previous doctor. They often express their
satisfaction with the first interview. Before long, they complain. Looking at the
pattern of their relationship with mental health services as a whole, it can appear
that complaint is the point of the exercise.

The complaints tend to be about minutiae or the intangible: that your manner
is wrong; that you are too critical or lack interest in them; that you are not
seeing them often enough or long enough. Sometimes there is a dispute over
the technical aspects of treatment: that you have the diagnosis wrong ('I've
been reading ICD 10. I haven't got a paranoid personality disorder, I've got an
obsessional personality disorder'); that you failed to warn about an infrequent
side effect that has now had an implausibly devastating effect on the patient's
life; or that you have misconstrued a part of the history to a third party.

One way of understanding these patients is that they have a profound belief
that no one cares about them and that they are helpless. They do not believe that
they can influence relationships and they do not expect that anyone will listen
or truly try to help them. They feel alone and neglected, and the complaints
are the angry consequence of this. Their unhappiness is experienced as being
autonomous, beyond their control and unrelated to their circumstances.
Even when they express initial scepticism about the doctor, they have an implicit
expectation that somewhere there is an ideal psychiatrist who can put things right

for them. The new doctor rapidly fails against this expectation, and the complaints start. The doctor becomes irritated or rejects them, confirming their beliefs about themselves and sustaining the cycle. Complaints and complaint systems create an opportunity to bring the existential unfairness of their lives to the attention of a wider audience.

In order to help these patients it is essential to break the pattern of movement between doctors. A further change solves your problem, but it does nothing for the patient or for your colleagues. A refusal to raise expectations may be useful, by stating at the start that you cannot promise to be any more helpful than the doctors that the patient has seen in the past. Sometimes a time limit for involvement leads to a negotiation over what might be realistically achieved in that time. A time limit avoids an indefinite struggle if it does not work out. Suggesting that realistically you are probably the last psychiatrist in the line can have a similar effect. All of this is easy when the pattern is long established, but a similar strategy can be employed when a pattern of complaint emerges after treatment has started. In all of this, one has to bear in mind the boy who cried wolf; even habitual complainers can have a good reason for complaint.

It can be possible to help these patients to achieve a more realistic understanding of their problems and to move on from the position of querulous helplessness; but not always.

Patients who threaten the doctor

Patients become threatening because they feel impotent within the relationship. They usually want something from the doctor that he is not prepared to give. This can include admission to hospital, or prescriptions of abusable drugs, or the provision of misleading information to another agency. Some patients threaten the doctor with violence, and many threaten to harm themselves or someone else, unless some unreasonable demand is met. These latter threats have a considerable impact in a world where psychiatrists are increasingly in fear of being held accountable for their patient's behaviour.

Threats of personal violence cannot be tolerated from patients who are not psychotic. If threats are persistent or acted upon, the police should always be involved. Aggressive people do not become less so if their actions are treated as inconsequential. Some patients persecute doctors, for example in the form of letters or phone calls. In these circumstances it is essential to inform your employers and take legal action promptly. The lack of a response to such activities can frustrate an ex-patient with a grudge and lead to an escalation of the harassment. Fortunately this occurs very rarely, but when it does you must protect yourself from it at an early stage.

Patients who threaten to harm themselves or other people are a difficult problem. Although many such patients are not mentally ill, some are. The problems they pose cannot be separated from issues of risk assessment. This is explored in Chapter 16.

A difficult interview

In the days before shift work, Dr Lee was the duty psychiatrist for a busy inner city Accident and Emergency Department (A&E). In the course of a particular evening, he assessed four patients. Two patients had to be admitted to hospital, which involved him in lengthy and frustrating telephone negotiations in order to find available inpatient beds. He finally went to bed himself at 1.30 am, only to be woken an hour later to assess yet another patient.

On arrival back in A&E, he was asked to see Mr Cox. Mr Cox turned out to be an angry 26-year-old man who was complaining of auditory hallucinations. He was demanding to be admitted to hospital. In the course of assessment, it emerged that he was living in a rough bed-and-breakfast hotel, and that he was a heavy drinker. He was in conflict with another resident, and was short of money; and it seemed likely to Dr Lee that he was concealing other factors relevant to his wish to be admitted.

Dr Lee could find no evidence that Mr Cox was seriously mentally ill. It was possible that he had alcoholic hallucinosis, but the complaints of hallucinations were vague and unconvincing. There were no other symptoms. It seemed quite clear that Mr Cox was at the end of his tether and saw admission to hospital as an available method of resolving his immediate problems.

Dr Lee was also a 26-year-old man at the end of his tether. He wanted to go to bed, and he was angered that he had to deal with an awkward patient who was not psychiatrically unwell. As the interview proceeded, the doctor and the patient became increasingly irritable with each other. Mr Cox was in difficulty. He did not know how to solve his problems, and his plan to become a psychiatric inpatient was not proceeding as he had hoped. Dr Lee was also in difficulty. If he admitted the patient he would be criticised the next day for the inappropriate use of a scarce resource. If he turned the patient away there might be unpleasantness.

The doctor and the patient were locked in a dysfunctional interaction, where their immediate problems mirrored each other. These situations are common, and the only way out of them is to recognise the nature of the dysfunction, which is that doctor and patient have a lot in common, but no common ground.

Dr Lee found a way forward. He pointed out that he was feeling tired and irritable, and that Mr Cox was probably feeling the same way. The interview was going nowhere because they had become locked in a struggle where neither could give way. There was no possibility of admitting Mr Cox. This was outside of his control. In any case, lying low in hospital would not make a blind bit of difference to Mr Cox's problems. They would be the same or worse on discharge. He acknowledged that Mr Cox had real and pressing difficulties, and discussed less immediate interventions that might ease Mr Cox's difficulties. The doctor and the patient were released from their conflict, and the next morning Dr Lee referred Mr Cox to a voluntary sector alcohol counselling service.

Such strategies do not always work. However, by offering the patient an alternative way forward the doctor at least feels less helpless and angry. This can, in turn, improve the dynamic with the patient.

This chapter has not attempted to exhaustively list all types of difficult interviews and unpopular patients. We have drawn out some themes that we find useful in dealing with difficult interviews. The main principles are robust over a wide range of problems. If they are observed, dysfunctional interactions can be avoided some of the time.

Main points in this chapter

1. In situations where the psychiatrist finds the patient difficult, there is usually a conflict between the doctor's and the patient's agendas.
2. Sometimes this has its origins in deep-seated attitudes and beliefs of the patient. We have called this the meta-agenda. It is often outside of the patient's awareness, but it determines more explicit agenda items.
3. If the psychiatrist attempts to force his agenda on the patient, the relationships will fail. It is better to search for a strategy that will establish common ground.
4. Setting limits, by being explicit about the length and objectives of treatment, and by establishing rules of conduct, is always helpful.
5. These patients are not necessarily impossible to help.

Part IV

Self-awareness

Psychiatry is an applied science. As such, objectivity is one of its central values and strengths. However, objectivity is not easily achieved, as the psychiatrist is far from neutral. This section is concerned with the impact of the mental health professional's personal characteristics as an active factor affecting interviews and assessment. This involves understanding how cultural difference, ideology and personality can affect evaluation of, and the relationship with, the patient. We all use our personalities and other individual characteristics as a clinical tool, but to do so we need to develop self-awareness.

9

Values and beliefs

In Chapter 6 we explored some problems and dilemmas that can arise within interactions between psychiatrists and patients. These factors, such as dependency, are part of the process of the therapeutic relationship. Here, we examine the impact of the professional's own values and beliefs upon the relationship.

We each have our individual, idiosyncratic, set of values and beliefs, but psychiatry itself contains values, determined by the social context from which it arises. No degree of abstraction can rid any science of its values. Absolute objectivity, in the sense of a God-like detachment, is impossible. This is not to deny that there are objective truths that exist independently of observers. The truth, however, is often complex. In psychiatry, we can only partially observe or explain behaviours, and it is inevitable that there is frequently more than one available partial explanation. This is not an excuse for abandoning the aim of objectivity. Objectivity is best served through an understanding of our own values and beliefs. Without this understanding, these values and beliefs can interfere in our clinical work.

Broadly speaking, values and beliefs operate at three distinct levels. Firstly, there are the values of the British medical profession. These subdivide into explicit, codified rules, set out as guidance by regulating bodies, and a more diverse, informal, set of shared ideas that constitute the medical subculture, within which there is a specifically psychiatric subculture.

Secondly, there is the individual's personal belief system, an explicit personal ideology that develops out of educational, class, family, religious and political backgrounds.

Finally, elements of personality shape implicit values, which may not be fully within the professional's awareness. These can make particular subjects or types of patients easier or more troublesome to deal with.

Medical values

From the time of Hippocrates, there was a perceived need to set out a code of values for doctors. The core values of British medicine were first formally set out by the General Medical Council (GMC) when it was formed in the nineteenth century. These values are generally liberal and rationalist, being broadly based upon the ideas of the Enlightenment. The code does change with time. For example, attitudes to termination of pregnancy have dramatically altered. The values behind the code arise through consensus. They are determined in part by leaders of the profession, in part by demands of the public and in part by governmental policy makers. The code is under revision at the time of writing, although it seems to us that there is a surprisingly high degree of agreement about it. Criticism of the profession, and calls for the abolition of the GMC, appear to be driven by the failure of the profession to adhere to the code at all times. The current formal code is set out in Box 9.1 (GMC, 2001).

BOX 9.1 The formal values of British medical practice (GMC, 2001)

Patients must be able to trust doctors with their lives and well-being. To justify that trust, we as a profession have a duty to maintain a good standard of practice and care and to show respect for human life. In particular as a doctor you must:

- make the care of the patient your first concern;
- treat every patient politely and considerately;
- respect patients' dignity and privacy;
- listen to patients and respect their views;
- give patients information in a way they can understand;
- respect the rights of patients to be fully involved in decisions about their care;
- keep your professional knowledge and skills up to date;
- recognise the limits of your professional competence;
- be honest and trustworthy;
- respect and protect confidential information;
- make sure that your personal beliefs do not prejudice your patients' care;
- act quickly to protect patients from risk, if you have good reason to believe that you or a colleague may not be fit to practice;
- avoid abusing your position as a doctor; and
- work with colleagues in ways that best serve patients' interests.

In all these matters, you must never discriminate unfairly against your patients or colleagues. Also, you must always be prepared to justify your actions to them.

The subcultures of medicine influence the formal code, but they can conflict with it and with each other. Significant groups of doctors hold values that, under some circumstances, are deviant and obstructive with regard to getting the job done. For example, there is intolerance in a proportion of the profession towards patients who are regarded as morally culpable for their own ill health. This can be directed at those with substance misuse problems, people who recurrently lacerate themselves, smokers with emphysema and so on. The problem with this attitude is not just that it is in conflict with the expectations of the formal code. Taking a position of moral condemnation also makes it more difficult to form relationships with such patients, to influence their behaviour and to help them to stop harming themselves.

Subcultural values do not belong to individuals. They are a group phenomenon. Consequently, well-meaning, and otherwise highly competent, individuals can hold values that are unhelpful or deviant. Deviant values tend to arise in groups that are inward-looking and isolated. This does not require geographical isolation. It can occur in tight-knit groups who work within larger organisations, such as general hospitals.

A very agitated 28-year-old woman burst into A&E one evening, demanding a brain scan. She was manic and had a delusion that she had a brain tumour. She was seen by a casualty officer, who tried to explain that a scan was not indicated. The patient rapidly became frustrated, and suddenly assaulted the doctor. He restrained her with the assistance of nursing staff, but, in the struggle, the patient bit him, breaking his skin. The patient was admitted to the psychiatric unit under legal compulsion.

Later that night, the casualty officer contacted the duty psychiatrist, asking that the patient be tested for HIV and hepatitis, so that he could find out whether he needed prophylaxis or not. The duty psychiatrist explained that the patient lacked mental capacity to consent to the tests, but in any case she was refusing all investigations. The casualty officer said that in A&E they took the view that, in assaulting staff, patients waived their rights. They had tested patients without consent under these circumstances in the past. Unable to reach agreement, the doctors handed the matter over to their consultants. The A&E consultant also pressed for the patient to be tested without consent, but the psychiatric consultant was not prepared to allow this. The conflict was resolved with discovery of specific guidance on the GMC web site, which stated that, to take blood or to carry out the tests without consent was both unlawful and unethical.

Variations in subcultural values between different parts of the profession are not necessarily a bad thing. For example, the degree of interpersonal engagement with patients that is prevalent amongst psychiatrists would be inappropriate in a surgeon. Psychiatrists are often very distressed when their patients die, and it is a shared subcultural value that this is appropriate. The same attitude would be very destructive in any branch of hospital medicine where death is a daily occurrence.

One of the strengths of medicine is that it does have an explicit code. This allows subcultural values to be measured for compatibility with society's expectations. This can occur only if one stays in touch with a wider body of opinion and debate. If one does not refer back to first principles, expedient solutions to tricky problems are likely to lead to trouble.

Personal ideology

Similar considerations apply to personal values and beliefs. Some people work in psychiatry because of deeply held personal beliefs, for example, a religious faith or a political commitment to the disadvantaged. For these professionals, there is no separation between their private values and their professional work. There is nothing wrong with this. However, these strong convictions can become a serious problem if the professional lacks self-awareness or is so convinced of his own belief system that he is prepared to proselytise, or otherwise force his ideas upon the patient.

Most psychiatrists have to bite their tongue from time to time. They have to put their own values to one side in the course of their work and decline to express strongly held views. However, this is not sufficient in itself to protect them from acting on their values. The trouble with deeply held beliefs is that people tend to experience them as universal truths. It takes a degree of self-discipline to monitor one's own behaviour and to ensure that decisions are not inappropriately affected by personal beliefs.

A GP referred a 30-year-old woman suffering from anxiety related to pregnancy. On assessment, it emerged that the woman was pregnant by a neighbour. Her husband knew nothing of the pregnancy, and she was desperate to terminate the pregnancy within the legal time limit. She had approached her GP, who, as a first step, had referred her to a 'pregnancy counsellor'. The counsellor turned out to be the GP's wife. Over a number of interviews, she had shown the patient photographs of foetuses, in order to help the patient to consider other options. On completion of counselling, she told her GP that she still wanted an abortion. He then explained that his religious beliefs prevented him from cooperating with the termination of a pregnancy, but that he was willing to send her for a psychiatric opinion.

The GP had the right to avoid actions that conflicted with his religious beliefs. He did not have the right to covertly impose his beliefs on the patient. His beliefs were affecting his professional behaviour, and he should have made this clear at the outset. He should have made it possible for the patient to see a different practitioner, no matter how wrong he felt that the outcome would be.

More subtle expressions of belief can also be damaging. For example, some people who do not recognise the legitimacy of the state of Israel refer to the geographical location as Palestine. However, to refer to Israel as Palestine to a Jewish patient is almost certain to raise an apprehension in the patient's mind about the doctor's attitude to Jews. Irrespective of the political arguments, to use such terminology is self-indulgent and abusive, as it serves the doctor's needs, not the patient's.

Strong convictions can lead to strong disapproval of some types of lifestyle. There are doctors who, if given the choice, would rather have nothing to do with racists, or homosexuals, or paedophiles. Such disapproval cannot be indulged. As a doctor, you either have to be prepared to treat everybody in the same way, or not to practice at all.

We all have ideas about how people should live, and these values can intrude into a wide range of clinical situations. The difference between a clinical judgement and a personal value can be quite ambiguous. For example, many psychiatrists, including ourselves, believe that the position of being a helpless victim is bad for people's mental health. Many doctors also abhor the compensation culture that has recently developed in the UK, not least because it has increased medical negligence litigation, and medical defence insurance premiums have risen. In discouraging a patient from engaging in a medical negligence claim against another doctor, is the psychiatrist protecting the patient from the victim role, or imposing his own values? There is not a simple answer to the question, but it is important that the psychiatrist should ask himself such questions.

All of these examples concern beliefs and values that are explicit. They are conscious and have a rationale. One could argue their merits. However, not all values and beliefs are like this.

Implicit values

There are some beliefs and values that are so deep-seated that we are hardly aware of them. They are rooted in our personality attributes and wider social attitudes. They cause problems through the intermediary of feelings of embarrassment or hostility towards patients.

For example, there is a social taboo against explicit discussion of sexuality with people of the opposite sex, and a further taboo against older people acknowledging that they are sexually active.

Mrs Thompson, a 47-year-old woman, has been referred by her GP. She sees Dr Nichol, a 26-year-old psychiatric trainee. On assessment, he finds that she is depressed. She makes a good recovery on a selective serotonin reuptake inhibitor (SSRI) antidepressant. At a follow-up appointment, she wishes to discontinue the medication because of side effects. Dr Nichol asks what side effects are bothering her. Mrs Thompson says that although the tablets have helped, she can no longer achieve orgasm and this is becoming a real problem.

Dr Nichol is acutely embarrassed. He does not want to discuss intimate details of the patient's sexual life. He is worried that any interest may appear prurient. He is very uneasy about discussing these matters with a much older woman.

Mrs Thompson has come to the interview expecting to discuss her sexual life. There was little point in raising the issue otherwise. Dr Nichol should explore the problem a little more before coming to a decision with the patient about what to do. The only obstruction to doing this is Dr Nichol's own values and inhibitions. He cannot stop himself from being uncomfortable by an act of will. Even after years of experience, some doctors remain uneasy talking with their patients about sexual matters. There is not an easy way around this. Sexual issues have to be discussed, whether the doctor is comfortable with it or not. If Dr Nichol acknowledges to himself that the problem is his, he stands a better chance of overcoming the difficulty. All forms of avoidance heighten anxiety; overcoming avoidance lessens it. Skirting around difficult subjects does not help much. Grasping the nettle and forcing oneself to break the taboo tends to work a lot better.

Values and beliefs can strongly colour expectations of patients with particular types of problems. Many doctors have very negative ideas about substance misusers, who are characterised as self-pitying, dishonest, manipulative and potentially aggressive. The doctor does not have to express such ideas for them to be a problem; they are bound to make him uncomfortable when interviewing substance misusers. He is hardly likely to be very helpful to these patients. On the other hand, some doctors feel no hostility towards substance misusers, but have a very narrow understanding of substance misusing lifestyles. This makes it difficult to obtain a substance misuse history, and ignorance can lead to an underestimation of the range of health problems caused by substance misuse. Alternatively, it can lead to the doctor inappropriately attributing all the patient's problems to substance misuse, thus missing independent treatable conditions.

It is impossible to practice psychiatry effectively unless one has the capacity to understand lifestyles different from one's own. For example, drugs are everywhere and all psychiatrists treat drug users. The only way of learning about the subject is either to immerse oneself in drug taking (a course that we do not recommend), or to learn from one's patients. Fixed stereotypes stand in the way of hearing what patients tell you. Prejudices can only be challenged if you acknowledge that you have them.

Paedophiles

If there is one group of people who really test psychiatrists' ability to rise above their personal values, it is paedophiles. Although many middle class professionals distance themselves from the modern witch-hunts and vigilante actions against paedophiles, generally they feel no more sympathy towards child-sex offenders than anyone else does. Paedophiles are the most vilified group in modern society, and most psychiatrists feel that this status is well-deserved.

It is not unusual for paedophiles to be referred to general psychiatrists. They sometimes have a suicidal crisis in the face of legal action. Sometimes they seek support for their claims that they are innocent victims of malicious accusations. Sometimes paedophiles develop mental illnesses that have little or nothing to do with their sexual behaviour. No one likes paedophilic sex offenders. They rarely like each other. They retain the loyalty of friends and family only by convincing them that they are innocent. Anyone who deals with paedophiles regularly knows that they are plausible liars. This creates a further dilemma, as some people accused of paedophilic offences are innocent, and become depressed as a consequence.

The strong negative feelings that paedophiles evoke are hard to overcome. One tends to have punitive feelings towards the offender, and the need to maintain a high degree of scepticism can be used to justify an inappropriately aggressive clinical approach. Paedophiles tend to have strong defences of rationalisation and denial. They often feel sorry for themselves and feel that they are the victim. The clinician experiences them as loathsome, self-pitying and self-justifying. Consequently, there is an understandable tendency to keep clinical involvement to a minimum. However, codified medical ethics insist that even paedophiles have a right to psychiatric treatment, if they genuinely need it. They have to be assessed as objectively as possible. Treatment of a psychiatric disorder occasionally reduces the risk of re-offending.

Mr Jones is a 32-year-old car mechanic. He is under investigation by social services and the police. His 7-year-old stepdaughter has told her grandmother that Mr Jones had intercourse with her when her mother was out. Medical examination has confirmed that intercourse has taken place. Mr Jones does not deny that the child has been abused, but he does deny that he is the abuser. The child has accused him, he claims, because he is stricter than the biological father. She has never accepted him as part of the household. His wife is convinced of his innocence, and as a consequence, the child has been taken by social services and placed in the care of her grandmother. Mr Jones is forbidden to have contact with her, and is not allowed to be alone with any other children. The family is in turmoil, and Mr Jones has approached his GP for psychiatric referral because he has been feeling desperate, and sometimes suicidal, over his situation.

Dr Coltrane has enough information from the referral letter to guess what has been going on. He does not like dealing with this type of situation. He is likely to face the assessment interview carrying a complex agenda. He wants to avoid colluding with the offender, and therefore cannot take Mr Jones' account at face value. He is bound to form a judgement as to whether the patient is or is not the abuser. As well as his responsibility to the patient, he has to bear in mind his responsibility to protect other children that Mr Jones may come into contact with. Within the interview, he aims to be neither obviously hostile, nor uncritically supportive. He has to contain his own feelings of revulsion. He needs to firmly control the interview. If Mr Jones needs treatment, he has to try to establish the basis for a therapeutic relationship. He will have to obtain information from social services before coming to a firm conclusion about the patient. He must consider the possibility that Mr Jones is telling the truth.

Inevitably, there is a further pitfall here. In trying to restrain one's antagonistic feelings towards a paedophile, it is possible to go too far. The clinician can effectively find himself in a state of denial, whereby he recognises that the patient is guilty of sexual offences against children, but puts this wholly outside of his awareness when dealing with the patient. This can easily lead to a situation in which the psychiatrist colludes with the paedophile, for example, by responding to a suicidal crisis by arranging a lengthy inpatient admission that delays a court case until it collapses.

The point of drawing out the problems in assessing people accused of paedophilic offences is that it is obvious that there is no simple solution to the strong feelings they evoke and the dilemmas in dealing with them. However, self-awareness does help, and can restrain the psychiatrist's most punitive instincts.

Main points in this chapter

1. All clinicians have values and beliefs that can interfere with therapeutic relationships.
2. Being aware of one's own implicit and explicit attitudes is helpful.
3. No matter how strong one's beliefs might be, all doctors have to work within the formal ethical code of medicine.

10

Culture

Culture is a configuration of belief, custom, language, social ritual, values and behaviour, which is held in common by a group of people who identify themselves as distinct from other groups. Culture is the most fundamental of our points of reference in life, and the filter through which we experience the world. However, within our own communities, we are hardly aware of our own culture. Generally speaking, we become conscious of our culture when it is contrasted with a different culture. In other words, we become aware that our cultural assumptions exist only when we meet someone who does not share them.

One of the strengths of modern inner cities is their vibrant cultural diversity. Most psychiatrists working in these areas become culturally aware and comfortable with working across cultural divides. That minority of psychiatrists who do not achieve this are of very limited use to their patients. Cultural awareness ultimately teaches you that different peoples have similar underlying needs. Cultural differences can be profound, but people are people. There is more that unites us than divides us.

Cultural awareness is harder to achieve when working with less diverse populations. It is often those mental health services that have the smallest number of patients from ethnic minorities that have greatest difficulty in dealing appropriately with cultural difference. Furthermore, culture is not synonymous with ethnicity. There are significant cultural differences between white middle class doctors and white working class patients. It can be hard to be aware of cross-class cultural differences.

Transcultural exotica versus cultural awareness

British psychiatry has intermittently become interested in 'culture bound syndromes'. For example, koro is said to be a manifestation of anxiety that occurs mainly amongst people in South Asia, particularly the Chinese. Koro is said to typically affect males. The victim suffers from somatic symptoms of anxiety, and becomes convinced that his penis is retracting into his body, and that this will kill him. Some sufferers try to stop or reverse the retraction process by tying a brick to their penis. There are a number of such culture bound syndromes.

The concept of the culture bound syndrome is not especially helpful. The extent to which such syndromes are bound to a single culture is far from clear. Koro has been reported in a wide variety of populations, including ethnic Europeans, and it can occur in women. There is a worrying implication that it is the bizarre and dramatic quality of koro that makes it interesting. There is an implied eurocentricity to the effect that Europeans have true mental disorders, whilst Africans and Asians have culture bound syndromes. There is a post-colonial anthropology here, an implicit suggestion that 'primitive peoples' lack sophistication, and that when they get anxious, they run around with bricks tied to their penises. Not only does this achieve nothing in helping individual patients, it also tends to obscure the true significance of culture, and the subtle ways in which culture shapes mental disorder.

Liverpool has the longest established Chinese community in Europe, and we have worked with this community over many years. Between us, we have only once ever seen a case of koro, and that affected an English teenager with no connection to the Chinese community. However, there are many cultural factors that do influence the presentation and treatment of mental illness in that community. These factors are complex, and generalisations can be misleading. Broadly speaking, there is a Chinese attitude that dictates that you should, as far as possible, avoid contact with authority; that you should cause no trouble and try to be invisible to officialdom. Chinese culture is stoical and uncomplaining. As a consequence, Chinese people tend to be deferential to doctors, and tend to want to be discharged from follow-up as quickly as possible. Chinese people tend not to press an understanding of their culture upon you; you have to actively seek to understand it.

The Chinese have a very different way, compared to Europeans, of understanding emotional and physical well-being. Concepts of balancing opposing influences, of yin and yang, are important. For example, they affect food and diet, which in any case have a particular role in social ritual. Psychotic experiences are often rationalised by the patient as being due to the influence of spirits or ancestors. However, whilst beliefs about spirits and ancestors are prevalent in the community, friends and family have little difficulty in distinguishing psychosis from more ordinary beliefs. Many Chinese people regard mental illness as shameful. The mentally ill are often intensively cared for by their family, and presentation to services tends to occur very late. People whose disturbed behaviour is loud, difficult and public can find themselves shunned and isolated. The Chinese community in Liverpool do not share a single language, the commonest tongues being Cantonese and Hakkar. Many women have only basic

English. Written Chinese pictograms, on the other hand, are not specific to a language, and are universally understood.

It is these types of cultural factors, rather than the exotic, which are worth knowing about, and which facilitate therapeutic relationships with patients from other cultures. You do, however, have to take the trouble to find out about minority communities.

Urban psychiatrists are likely to deal with patients who speak a wide range of languages, and come from diverse cultures. It would be impossible to have prior knowledge of all of these. All psychiatrists have to use translators from time to time, and have to be prepared to understand something of the patient's culture by asking directly about it (Box 10.1).

BOX 10.1 Not all differences are cultural in origin

Dr Holliday is a GP. She is called out at night by a couple to see their 5-year-old son. The couple came to the UK from India a year ago. They are very polite, and obviously relieved to see the doctor. The child is mildly pyrexial, complains of generalised aches and pains, and has a sore throat. He is not unduly distressed, and the only physical finding is inflamed fauces. Dr Holliday is annoyed. The child clearly has a mild viral infection that does not merit a home visit at night. She is tempted to reprimand the family for abusing her availability, but she is curious as to why the parents are so worried. She asks them what they had thought was wrong with the child. They reply that they feared he had rheumatic fever. Rheumatic fever is common in India and it is a major cause of morbidity. Sore throat, joint pains and pyrexia are the presenting symptoms. Their anxiety is reasonable and understandable.

Working with translators

The use of translators is essential wherever the patient's first language is not spoken English (even where the person has some English). The difference between interpreters and translators is that interpreters bring an element of analysis and explanation to the task. In psychiatry, interpretation is less satisfactory than translation, because the interpreter unwittingly usurps the psychiatrist's role by trying to make sense of things. However, translation is also problematic. Even the best translators have difficulty in conveying the subtleties and nuances of what is being said. Professional translators are generally better than family or friends. Professional translators are taught to avoid interpreting too much, to avoid organising and thus altering what is said. Family and friends almost always have their own agenda, and, of course, confidentiality is compromised. However, professional translators usually come from the patient's own community, and are likely to be directly or indirectly known to the patient. This can create real problems. Telephone translation services can get round this, but they are slow and cumbersome to use (Box 10.2).

BOX 10.2 A translation problem

Mrs Khan is a 55-year-old Pakistani lady. She is referred by her GP to be seen at home by Dr Coltrane. She has taken to bed over the past two months and she will not get up. She is reluctant to eat and her GP thinks she is depressed. Mrs Khan lives with her husband and their extended family in a Victorian terraced house. She speaks no English.

Dr Coltrane is greeted by Mrs Khan's eldest son, who was born in the UK. He explains that his father, who also speaks little English, would like to have a few words before his wife is seen. The elder Mr Khan, using his son as translator, explains that his wife is complaining of weakness, and that she is suffering from a headache. He is worried because it is unusual for her to be ill.

Dr Coltrane goes to the bedroom, which is rather bare. Mrs Khan is huddled under the bedclothes, and she is moaning quietly. Again, using the younger Mr Khan as translator, he tries to interview Mrs Khan. Her answers are brief. After twenty minutes, he is not getting very far. He begins to wonder why she is so reluctant to tell him anything, and asks 'Is anyone frightening you?' Mrs Khan is momentarily more animated, speaking and gesturing at some length. Her son translates: 'No'. It is obvious to Dr Coltrane that whatever Mrs Khan said, it was more complicated than 'No'. He presses her son to tell him exactly what she said. He replies that she had said no, and that the rest of the answer was rubbish. Further pressed, he looks embarrassed and laughs uncomfortably. He reveals that Mrs Khan had complained that there are Germans on the roof who talk about her constantly and prevent her from sleeping. Her son takes pains to point out that this is patently untrue. Insisting that all further translation is verbatim, Dr Coltrane slowly elicits a range of psychotic phenomena.

There are some broad principles which are helpful when working with translators (including sign language translators):

1. It is better to postpone an interview than to go ahead with an inadequate or inappropriate translator. Delay is usually less of a problem than getting things wrong.
2. Translators need to be told to translate exactly what has been said in each direction, and where this is difficult, to ask the speaker to rephrase what they have said.
3. Before the interview commences, make sure that the patient is comfortable with the translator.
4. As far as possible, avoid using family and friends as translators.

5. Do not interview the translator. Look at the patient as you normally would in an interview.

6. Try to keep sentences short, and avoid both jargon and colloquial forms of expression.

7. In the course of any translation, some responses to questions will be muddled. It is important to clarify these, to be clear whether the muddle is linguistic or a reflection of the patient's mental state.

8. When conveying information to the patient, say it at least twice in different ways, and ask that he repeats back what he has been told.

9. At the end of the interview, it is worth asking the translator for his impression, as at that stage he can safely *interpret* what has been said, and explain cultural nuances.

Cross-class subcultural differences

Communities are not geographical entities. They are groups of people who interact sufficiently frequently to develop a sense of cohesion. In both towns and the countryside, communities exist alongside each other, often with little contact or mutual awareness. In the UK, class is a particularly strong subculture, around which communities form. However, lifestyle can carry the same function. A gay subculture and community exists (though not all gay people live within it). Many homeless people live in city centres close to the hub of society's financial and political institutions, with a lifestyle and subculture that is utterly alien to the mainstream of British society.

Homelessness has a very strong association with mental disorder, be it mental illness, substance dependency or personality disorder. It is hard to know whether a significant proportion of single homeless people were ever stereotypical tramps, but they certainly are not now. The middle-aged street drinker, dishevelled and shouting, may use homeless facilities, but they often have accommodation. They gravitate to street drinking because they are not tolerated in pubs.

Homeless people tend to be young and white. The only ethnic minority with significant representation amongst the homeless is the Irish. Young homeless people tend to have a background history of family disturbance, and of growing up in local authority care. Some become homeless when they leave the armed forces. Very few live permanently on the streets. They tend to have unstable accommodation, moving between hostels, bed-and-breakfast establishments, bondies (empty buildings), prison and the streets. Most have problems that lead to antisocial behaviour, and exclusion because of this behaviour drives the instability in their living circumstances. Drug and alcohol misuse is often a primary activity, and this necessitates criminality and prostitution. Exploitation and manipulation of the settled population is an accepted social norm. Although homeless environments are violent and dangerous, homeless people maintain high levels of co-operation, and tend to look after each other. Their decision-making can appear short sighted, but looking after immediate needs is more important than worrying about long-term concerns when you are living under extreme conditions. The degree of mutual support and comradeship in homelessness can make it very difficult to settle in more isolated permanent accommodation, and some people choose to return to the streets. It can be hard for middle class professionals to understand that, despite the deprivation and squalor of homelessness, the lifestyle has some advantages for some people.

Racism

One of the difficulties about being a member of an ethnic minority in the UK is that there is a significant chance of being the victim of racism. This does not affect all ethnic minorities and individuals to the same extent. However, it is hard to deny that racism is a tangible reality in the everyday lives of a significant proportion of the ethnic minority population.

Racism is a complex phenomenon. Some elements are ideological and explicit. They involve direct threats to people's well-being, such as racial harassment and racially motivated violence. Other elements are implicit and unspoken, and they may be invisible to white people. Examples include the experience of young black men at the hands of the criminal justice system, barriers to employment, and difficulties in securing appropriate housing. Racial tensions exist between different ethnic minorities, and this too may be outside of the awareness of the majority community.

Racism can be an important part of the context in which black people become mentally ill, and the problems it causes have to be understood. Psychiatrists need to be prepared to acknowledge that racism is a tangible reality. There is little point in helping someone to recover from a mental illness as an inpatient, if they are to return to a housing situation where they are constantly racially harassed, as they are unlikely to remain well under such circumstances.

Black patients sometimes accuse individual psychiatrists of being racist. Few psychiatrists regard themselves as racist, and many identify themselves as anti-racists. The accusation may seem tiresome and groundless, and even offensive. It is hard to form a positive relationship with someone who assumes that you are prejudiced against them from the start. The accusation most commonly arises in the context of the psychiatrist detaining the patient against their will, or making some other unwelcome decision. To the psychiatrist, his actions clearly have nothing to do with ethnicity or racism. However, it is understandable that, if you experience racism in your daily life, you are likely to interpret incomprehensible and unwelcome professional behaviour in the same terms. Understanding this makes it easier to build a therapeutic relationship later.

Just to complicate things, there is racism within mental health services. Our organisations do not stand separate from the rest of society, and there is no reason to expect that health services will be any more or less racist than any other British institution. Some individual members of staff hold racist beliefs. There are many ethnic minority staff working within the mental health services, but they are disproportionately concentrated in low status jobs. In trying to get past the patient's perception that he may be a racist, the psychiatrist is at a disadvantage if there is obvious evidence of racism in his working environment.

This is not to say that all black patients approach services with an agenda dominated by suspicion and an expectation of racism. We are not recommending that psychiatrists treat people from ethnic minorities any differently from the rest of the population. Indeed, most would be very happy to be treated the same as anyone else. The point is to accept and to understand that issues of racism are important. They are distinct from issues of culture.

Special minorities

There are some minorities who have problems beyond those of cultural difference and racism. They experience special forms of marginalisation. A long period of liberal consensus about ethnicity, cultural diversity and migration has ended. Xenophobia has returned as part of the mainstream political discourse. This has left some populations struggling with new and severe problems.

The concept of the 'asylum seeker' is relatively new. It was developed as a deliberate policy in order to create an alternative to the term 'refugee', which evokes general sympathy. It is tied to the concept that a large proportion of refugees have no genuine fear of persecution at home and attempt to enter the UK either to find work or to claim benefits. This does not correspond with our experience from working with refugees. Whether or not one is sympathetic to 'asylum seekers', there can be little doubt about the consequences of government policy towards them. They are given very little cash. They are compelled to live in particular places, often 'dispersal centres' in provincial cities. They are prevented from settling into national groupings, so they are frequently very

> **BOX 10.3 Not all problems have a satisfactory solution**
>
> Dr Omatayo is a Nigerian psychiatrist who has been working in a UK university department for a year. He is an experienced doctor with a postgraduate qualification in psychiatry. He is working abroad to complete his training, but he is employed as an SHO, which is a post of lower status than the one that he occupied at home. On his first evening on call in A&E, a 24-year-old white man is brought in by the police, having been found walking along the central reservation of a dual carriage way. He is agitated and shouting, and he has hit a policeman on the way to hospital.
>
> When Dr Omatayo enters the room, the man spits at him. He then breaks into a rapid and unbroken tirade that is extremely offensive. Neither the police nor the doctor can interrupt or make him listen to any questions. The man makes many racist references to Dr Omatayo, and he complains that Dr Omatayo has been having sex with white nurses outside of the consulting room door. He condemns the police for interfering with English people when they should be sending blacks back to their own country. He says that if the police leave, the doctor will castrate him, and he demands to see a solicitor about being forced to see a black doctor.
>
> Dr Omatayo is very shaken by what the man is saying, and by his inability to control the interview. The policemen ask him to leave because, they say, his presence is making the man more aggressive and they fear that he will become assaultive.
>
> Dr Omatayo is now in a dilemma. He has no previous experience of open racism. He is uncertain whether the man is expressing unpleasant but genuinely held views (that is, the man is an ideological racist) or whether the man is simply very psychotic. The nursing staff are outraged and feel he should not have to put up with this abuse. They suggest that the police should be allowed to take the patient to the police station in order to charge him for the previous assault. What should he do?

isolated. They can be moved at short notice. They are condemned in the press, and harassed by local people. If they are refused asylum, they have no means to support themselves, and are required to return to their country of origin. A significant number have experienced torture and other trauma. Some of them develop acute mental illness. It is hard to overcome the combined effects of displacement, impoverishment, communication problems, vilification, traumatisation and insecurity. Working with asylum seekers creates significant practical, clinical and ethical problems.

There is a parallel with the situation of travellers or 'gypsies'. Although gypsies were subject to genocide by the Nazis, open prejudice against them remains acceptable in British society. Rural pubs sometimes have signs at the door saying 'No travellers'. Although not necessarily poverty stricken, travellers live quite separate lives, marked by frequent changes of location. Travellers experience real difficulties in accessing services such as education and health care.

They are generally perceived as intrinsically criminal, and can be subject to severe harassment.

Offering even basic mental health services to asylum seekers and travellers is difficult. It demands that mental health professionals make special efforts to understand the lives, culture and problems of people who are generally vilified. They rarely receive treatment of the same quality as that offered to the rest of the population. In the face of our frank inability to offer a solution to this, we suggest that an awareness of these problems is valuable (Box 10.3).

Main points in this chapter

1. Ultimately, notwithstanding cultural differences, nearly everyone in the world wants and needs the same things.
2. The effects of cultural difference can create problems for the psychiatrist, but they are not impossible to overcome.
3. Racism is a social reality that cannot be ignored.
4. Not all problems have solutions. The effects of cultural difference, racism and social marginalisation can make it impossible to offer people an equivalent service to that offered to the rest of the population, but the effort is worthwhile.

11

Who should I be?

Your clinical persona can only draw upon your personality. You cannot successfully develop a wholly contrived psychiatric persona, because the outcome is bound to be affected and uncomfortable. Indeed, the quality of *authenticity* is invaluable, and it is more important than any other individual personal characteristic. It is natural that patients find it easier to trust psychiatrists who seem relaxed, genuine and engaging. There are some other personal qualities that are desirable. These qualities are evident in naturally talented mental health professionals from the day they start training. The rest of us have to cultivate these qualities, which is perfectly possible, as long as you know what they are.

Psychological mindedness

Psychological mindedness has a particular meaning in psychotherapy, but it also has a more general meaning. It has little to do with the science of psychology. It concerns an ability to think about behaviour in terms of people's emotional lives. It is the ability to empathically understand how people feel, to understand 'what makes them tick'. People who are psychologically minded are good at predicting how other people will behave. They can imagine what it is like to be someone else, and how alien emotions can affect behaviour. In many ways, psychological mindedness is the opposite of narcissism, where other people are not understood as being fully autonomous, but are experienced as servants of the narcissist's needs.

People who are psychologically minded observe people all the time, not just at work. They notice patterns of interaction and make connections between emotional themes. When they cannot understand other people's behaviour, they generate a range of theories to explain it.

Curiosity and an ability to understand other lifestyles

The curiosity about other people that is useful in a psychiatrist goes beyond ordinary social interest. It verges on the psychologically prurient. It is an intense interest in other people's biographies and in the ways in which they experience the world. The process of finding out about other people is closely linked to imagining what it must be like to be them, out of which springs an understanding of their lifestyle. Curiosity about other people's lifestyles and life histories goes hand-in-hand with psychological mindedness. It is this curiosity that provides the information to develop psychological mindedness.

Warmth and a non-judgemental attitude

To be a psychiatrist you have to like people. Not everyone does. Some people prefer animals, or motor cars, or computers. Psychiatrists encounter patients from a very wide range of backgrounds. They often disapprove of, or are shocked by, their patients' lifestyles. However, they are not employed to make their patients into better people. They are employed to help them overcome mental health problems, and this is difficult if the therapeutic relationship is affected by disapproval or an emotional coldness. Warmth is important to all therapeutic relationships. This is not to say that psychiatrists should be emotionally gushing, hugging their patients and creating friendships with them. The degree of warmth in the relationship has to be compatible with maintaining boundaries. The psychiatrist has to remain capable of making dispassionate and objective judgements. The use of warmth in the relationship is in fact somewhat contrived, in that it is deliberately cultivated to achieve a specific end.

The term 'non-judgemental' is a little misleading. It means that the use of warmth is tempered by a type of neutrality. To be neutral does not imply being entirely uncritical. It is necessary to find a position that is neither censorious nor collusive. This type of neutrality means, for example, that when a male psychiatrist is treating a female prostitute, she feels comfortable in talking about her lifestyle and she feels that the psychiatrist thinks no less of her than of any other woman. However, it must be possible for the psychiatrist to discuss with his patient, at the right moment, the effect that prostitution is having on her self-esteem and emotional well-being.

Unflappability

Temperamentally anxious psychiatrists tend to make patients feel worse and spread panic amongst mental health teams. In clinical work, the unexpected happens regularly. One of the real challenges of psychiatry is that, no matter how experienced you are, you continue to face novel situations and have extremely difficult decisions to make. It is important to maintain the appearance of calmness and to rise above one's own fears, in order to make well thought through decisions. Unflappability does not imply that one does not get anxious. Indeed, blasé and complacent psychiatrists are dangerous. However, you cannot indulge yourself in regularly appearing panicky.

Tolerance of uncertainty

Psychiatry is full of uncertainty. You rarely know whether a decision has been a good one until long after it has been made. Plans to contain risk are often compromises and they have flaws. Sometimes it takes months or years to properly understand a patient, and you have to make decisions in the interim, in the face of uncomfortable ambiguities. If a psychiatrist finds it difficult to tolerate uncertainty, this is likely to cause problems to him and his patients. He is likely to find the job unpleasantly stressful, or he will cause significant problems by trying to introduce certainty where none exists, or, most likely, both. No one is entirely comfortable in the face of uncertainty, but you have to learn to put up with it.

Ability to maintain boundaries

Some mental health professionals have a good understanding of where professional boundaries lie, but they break them anyway. This is often a recurrent pattern. It usually has its origins in a personal need, a kind of neurotic craving to fulfil personal emptiness that overrides professional taboos. Professional boundaries have to be profound principles, rules that are constantly in your awareness. Incipient breaches need to ring alarm bells. Maintenance of boundaries needs to be automatic and effortless. If this does not happen, therapeutic relationships are bound to go wrong.

Streetwise

Everyone seems to agree that being streetwise is an invaluable asset to a psychiatrist. No one, however, seems to be able to define quite what it is, or how to develop it. It relates to a particular kind of knowingness, a sensitive awareness of some of the tough realities of life as it is lived. It is the quality that allows some people to read a situation, to know that it is unsafe to walk down a particular street on a particular day, where a less worldly colleague would obliviously stroll on and get mugged. It allows some people to easily spot dissimulation and lying, and to recognise a scam. It is not the same as cynicism. Streetwise psychiatrists have better relationships with patients living on the margins of society, because the patient comes to recognise that the psychiatrist understands his world. Unfortunately, being streetwise seems to be innate, not learned.

What am I getting out of this?

The general social attitude towards mental illness remains one of fear and ignorance. A medical degree opens up many career opportunities, and no one is forced to work as a psychiatrist. We make a choice to work in an arena that other people shun. It seems likely that there is something unusual about psychiatrists that makes us want to work with mental illness. It is as well to understand what this is. This is not to say that our motivations are pathological. On the contrary, they are inevitable, and are only likely to cause problems if we fail to understand them. It is only possible to offer an illustrative, rather than an exhaustive, list. They include:

Personal experience of mental illness

A significant proportion of psychiatrists have witnessed mental illness in someone close to them, usually a family member, during their early life. A smaller number have been seriously mentally unwell themselves. This is not surprising. Many health professionals are drawn to their careers after personal experience of serious illness. For some psychiatrists there is a powerful need to understand mental illness. One can speculate, for example, that this is an attempt to resolve the confusion and fear generated by living with a mentally ill relative. Such motivations can run out of control. For example, heroic and excessive efforts to try to rescue patients from their own behaviour can follow the failure to rescue someone in one's personal life. On the other hand, some psychiatrists seem to strip mental illness of its emotional content through an excessively reductionist approach. Mental illness becomes nothing more than a dry formula of neurotransmitter dysfunction or automatic negative cognitions (though neither biological psychiatry nor CBT are intrinsically reductionist or emotionless). If you have experienced mental illness as incoherent and frightening in your personal life, it may be comforting to conceptualise it in a more logical and emotionless way. The penalty may be an impairment of empathy and rapport with patients.

Psychological voyeurism

Some people with severe mental illness exist at the outer limits of human experience. Psychiatrists regularly encounter situations that are outlandish and bizarre. Working as a psychiatrist is often stressful, but it is rarely boring. The work offers unrivalled opportunities for voyeuristic excitement. Psychiatry opens a window on the most hidden aspects of life, and it would be foolish to deny that this is attractive to a lot of psychiatrists.

Related to voyeurism is a fascination with the intellectual puzzle at the heart of psychiatry. The basic nature of mental illness is a scientific, philosophical and social conundrum, which allows endless debate, controversy and theorising. Each patient's problem is a smaller puzzle. Many psychiatrists enjoy the cerebral challenge of their work.

Voyeurism can boil over, and excitement over the bizarre can obstruct an interest in helping the person. Voyeurism can be rationalised into, for example, an interest in psychopathology or rare syndromes. Patients can become 'a really amazing case of …'. Psychiatry is for patients, not for psychiatrists, and excessive voyeuristic or cerebral interest can reverse this.

Fantasies of omnipotence

Psychiatrists do have extensive legal powers over patients. Their opinions are treated with great respect by important social institutions such as the courts. Very unwell patients often make remarkable recoveries as a consequence of treatment. Despite negative stereotypes and a low status within medicine, psychiatrists do wield enormous social power. There is real potential for narcissistic pleasure, and for the psychiatrist to come to feel that he is more than an ordinary human being. A cult of personality can develop around charismatic psychiatrists, and this can allow them to become isolated, idiosyncratic and ultimately deviant. Some less charismatic psychiatrists are alone in their omnipotent fantasies, and their teams come to despise them.

Vicarious care receiving

Teenage motherhood has a number of causes. It tends to occur in needy, emotionally deprived young women who find vicarious fulfilment of their emotional needs through looking after a helpless but emotionally responsive infant. An attenuated form of this dynamic is widespread in the 'caring professions'. Looking after other people is not just pleasurable because of their gratitude; it often has an element of vicariously meeting a personal need to be involved in a caring relationship. This sort of vicarious care-receiving through care-giving is based on a type of projective identification. It is hardly surprising that it is common in psychiatry, where the degree of emotional engagement with patients is unusually high.

Pseudo-altruism

Community psychiatry is a form of social medicine, as are general practice and community paediatrics. Severe mental illness is a disease of poverty in much the same way that tuberculosis is a disease of poverty. Anyone can get it, but by and large, poor people do. Psychiatrists tend to work with a stigmatised and deprived population. A desire to champion and help the underdog, a kind of missionary fervour, attracts some doctors to psychiatry. This is a form of pseudo-altruism, as it serves the doctor's need to do good, which is often linked to strong political or religious convictions. This can turn into a self-righteous campaigning zeal, where the doctor's interests and the patients' interests become blurred, and personal axes are ground in the guise of advocacy.

Displacement of emotional distress

In a therapeutic relationship, the patient is the one with the illness, and recognising this guards a number of boundaries. Patients and professionals, however, do not belong to separate categories of humanity. Health professionals of all types are prone to lose sight of this and to feel that illness happens to patients; that they are protected because they are professionals. Mental health staff can experience serious mental distress in others, whilst feeling personally invulnerable. Confronted with distressing circumstances in their personal lives, they adopt an intellectualising, unemotional persona, which can be very mal-adaptive. Their work allows them to displace emotion away from themselves, but there is a penalty. When they do become depressed or otherwise mentally unwell, they are very reluctant to accept help.

Main points in this chapter

1. There is no ideal clinical persona for a psychiatrist. You can only build on who you actually are.
2. There are, however, some broad characteristics which are helpful, and which can be cultivated.
3. All mental health professionals serve some personal needs through their work. There is a range of motivations for being a psychiatrist, none of which are intrinsically pathological, but all of which can cause problems if they run out of control.

Part V

Out of the clinic

In modern practice, assessments and interviews are frequently conducted outside of the traditional one-to-one clinic model. Multidisciplinary assessment, interviews with informants and families, and interviews in patients' homes are essential elements of clinical practice. This is particularly the case in the treatment of people suffering from more serious mental illness. These ways of working can provide a richer, more accurate, assessment. They can lay the foundations of a more constructive relationship with the patient and can facilitate the development and implementation of complex care plans. However, they also introduce complexities and novel dilemmas.

12

Interviewing with other team members

Multidisciplinary interviewing is not a recent innovation. The traditional mental hospital weekly ward round was a form of multidisciplinary interview, though it was often poorly conducted. A large group of professionals, some of them unknown to the patient, held interviews that were dominated by one group of professionals, psychiatrists. Introductions were unusual, and the purpose of the interview was rarely explained to the patient, who had to work it out for himself. The rules of the interview were obscure, and it was easy to humiliate the patient, who was at a severe disadvantage compared with the professionals. Most patients hated ward rounds as a consequence. Like everything else, multidisciplinary interviewing can also be misused.

Even taking this into account, there are a number of circumstances where joint interviews have significant advantages:

- Different disciplines bring different perspectives and skills to interviews. Joint assessment interviews have a stereoscopic quality that can lead to a greater depth of understanding and better assessment.
- Patients with serious mental illnesses and complex needs are likely to benefit from the involvement of more than one type of professional in their care. It makes little sense to put patients through multiple assessments and reviews if this can be avoided. Where disciplines do interviews together, coordination and consistency of treatment is improved, and decision-making can be truly shared.
- A team member sometimes needs help from a different discipline to resolve a problem in the patient's care. For example, a community nurse might need a psychiatrist to help resolve a problem with medication side effects. One-off consultations are difficult if the team member who needs advice is not present in the room. It is usually best, and most practical, for these interviews to be carried out by the professionals together. This ensures that the problem has been properly dealt with, that the solution is appropriate to the overall situation, and that there have been no misunderstandings.

Although there are considerable advantages to joint interviewing in terms of the quality of assessment and efficient use of time, the presence of two professionals does have a major impact on the patient. Many, if not most, patients regard different individuals and professionals within a team in rather different ways. Relationships with nurses tend to be more informal than relationships with doctors. Doctors tend to be experienced as more intimidating than social workers. This means that patients often trust some members of the team more than others.

The presence of a trusted professional can greatly enhance an interview. For example, people with schizophrenia often come to know their community mental health nurse extremely well, and place great trust in them. Psychiatrists, on the other hand, tend to be more remote and formal. No matter how pleasant the psychiatrist may be, being interviewed by him can be daunting for the patient. Patients often value the support of their community nurse during the interview. The interview is less affected by the patient's apprehensions. The community nurse is likely to be able to bring problems to light that would otherwise have gone unmentioned. The nurse, the psychiatrist and the patient can hold a three-way discussion about problems and plans.

It can, however, go wrong. The intended threesome can split into two conflicting camps. If the patient does not trust either team member, he can feel bullied by the two professionals. If the team members do not have a good relationship, the interview can become a struggle between them. The patient and the nurse together can end up feeling browbeaten by the psychiatrist. Patients can feel inhibited from discussing sensitive subjects when there are two professionals in the room. They can develop worries about confidentiality. There is more to successful joint interviews than simply putting three people in a room together and hoping for the best.

Team work and team culture

Joint interviews are difficult to conduct if the two team members do not know each other well. Consultant psychiatrists work with a single team for many years, and team-working becomes second nature. Team members get to know one another's idiosyncrasies. Over many joint interviews, a joint style develops organically, by trial and error, on the basis of what works. The longer you are a member of a team, the more you affect team culture, and the more comfortable working within that culture becomes.

The problem for psychiatric trainees is that they change jobs frequently. They are constantly getting to know other team members. Team culture varies enormously between teams within the same organisation. Patterns of authority and status do not always conform to job descriptions. Working practices are often very different because of individual preferences or differences in patient populations.

The psychiatric trainee is often the least experienced member of the team, and the person least familiar with joint interviewing. Nonetheless, because of professional roles, other team members may look to the trainee to lead joint interviews. It is important as well to learn to adjust to unfamiliar working environments as quickly as possible. This requires observation and modelling. Team members lose sight of the idiosyncrasies in their working practices. They forget that teams work differently to each other. They are not well placed to recognise what a newcomer needs to know. The best way to learn about joint interviewing is to let a more experienced professional take the lead, even if this cuts across professional status.

People with well-developed skills always make complicated tasks look easy, and highly structured activities look casual and ad hoc. This is why experienced clinicians can appear to effortlessly resolve previously intractable problems. To the experienced, the structure of joint interviewing is so self-evident that they are hardly aware that they are following it.

Planning the interview

The key to successful joint interviewing is planning. Where both team members know each other and the patient well, this may require no more than a few moments of discussion just before the interview. Under other circumstances it may require a good deal more preparation than this. No matter how pressed for time you may be, it is always best to have a pre-interview discussion.

Collation of information

Case notes, no matter how well maintained, rarely hold all the relevant information. In any case, it is difficult to extract information from records quickly, and to separate the relevant from the trivial. In any case team members often have a far more detailed and sophisticated knowledge of the patient than is recorded in the notes. It is advisable to take some time to go over the information that is held by each of you, and to be clear about the reliability, or otherwise, of the information you have. If nothing else, this will ensure that you are both up to date and working on the same information.

Purpose and duration of the interview

It is always a good idea to be clear as to why you are seeing a patient, but it is particularly important that team members should have a shared understanding of the purpose of a joint interview. It may be that the interview is a routine review, and that the role of the psychiatrist is simply to hear that things are going well. If he does not know this at the outset, he may be more easily tempted into changing things. Interviews aimed at resolving medication problems, assessing suicide risk or reconsidering diagnosis, each require a different emphasis. The team members should try to agree a basic agenda for the interview, establishing those matters that each of them want covered before it is over. They need to agree upon a maximum duration for the interview.

Roles

Finally, there should be an agreement as to who will take the lead in the interview, and who will keep notes. Sometimes both parties have to keep notes. Doctors in the UK cannot delegate note keeping to non-medical staff and are expected to keep a record of all clinical interviews.

The interview

Before the interview starts you should ensure that the patient knows who the professionals are, and why they are at the interview. This may involve an explanation of an unfamiliar role. Often, it is helpful to state the purpose of the interview as agreed between the team members.

Generally speaking the main focus should be on the agreed lead interviewer, who should periodically invite the other interviewer's observations or comments. The other interviewer may want to ask further questions or to take over, and needs to be given an opportunity to do so. This avoids one interviewer breaking into a dialogue and disrupting it. Patients are sometimes keen to talk to the other interviewer, in which case one should adapt to their preference.

Experienced joint interviewers often use the technique of dialogue between the two professionals. This can be useful under a range of circumstances, and seeks to draw the patient into the professionals' way of understanding the situation. It is not an especially easy technique to master. There is a risk of patronising, or alienating, the patient. It is probably best reserved for use where the team members know each other well.

Breaks in joint interviews can be helpful, especially where things are not going well. They allow discussion between the interviewers and, where necessary, can help to refocus the interview. When difficult decisions have to be made, for example, as to whether a patient should be legally detained, such breaks are essential. They allow interviewers to make sure that they agree, and to make plans on what to do if the patient reacts badly to the conclusion of the interview. Such breaks do not arise in one-to-one interviews, and at first it can feel unnatural to suggest a break. In fact patients often welcome a break and a cup of tea, and, where the interview has become tense, a break can defuse the situation.

Debriefing

Generally speaking, there should be a brief discussion between the team members after the interview. This allows impressions to be shared, agreement on how secure any conclusions are and the identification of remaining gaps in information. It also allows feedback between team members on joint interviewing technique.

Main points in this chapter

1. Joint interviewing has significant advantages, but it can also be intimidating for patients.
2. Planning the interview is essential.
3. One person should lead the interview.
4. Breaks for discussion are useful when interviews run into difficulties.

13

Interviewing families and other informants

The ability to conduct successful interviews with patients' families and friends is a fundamental psychiatric skill. However, theoretical aspects of family interviewing are drawn mainly from family therapy, and can be dauntingly complex. There are several distinct family therapies (for example, systemic, behavioural and structural), which use different approaches to family interviewing. Psychiatrists need a small repertoire of generic family interviewing skills in order to confidently conduct routine family and informant interviews. Experience builds skills, and family theory is far more useful to the experienced interviewer than to the beginner. This chapter is concerned with the basics of family interviewing.

The main reasons for routine family interviewing are:

- To gather information about the patient that they are unable to give themselves, and to verify certain types of information.
- To have a dialogue with the family about the nature of the mental illness, about treatment plans and to discuss what they can do to help.
- To assess relationships and overall family functioning.
- To assess the impact of the patient's illness and behaviour on those around him, especially on carers and children.
- To establish and maintain a relationship whereby professionals and family can work together to help the patient.

Doctors have a tendency to regard talking with families as a chore that is a distraction from the main task of treatment. Psychiatry on the other hand has a marked tendency to locate the causes of mental illness within the family. Genetics, child abuse and high expressed emotion, for example, are all primarily family phenomena. Irrespective of the contribution that such factors may make to mental ill health, families and friends are important in patients' lives. Professionals are transient figures, but families are forever. No matter how far one might migrate socially or geographically, no one can escape the internalised influence of one's family of origin. It is important that mental health services be able to work positively with families, irrespective of whether one approves of their lifestyle or not.

Families and friends have their own needs, and they are often profoundly affected by the patient's condition. This can make family interviews highly charged and emotional, and there is a real risk of conflict with the clinician. It can be hard to follow the discussion because different family members have different opinions, and because of habitual patterns of family interaction. Protecting boundaries can be difficult, as families may not see why they are important. Families sometimes come to interviews with an agenda dominated by a desire to influence the professional's assessment of the patient, or a wish to influence decision-making in order to achieve a particular outcome. The family and the clinician can end up taking rhetorical positions that cannot be reconciled.

It can sometimes be helpful to think of families as systems, rather than just as groups of individuals. Some ideas that we have found helpful are set out in Box 13.1.

Before the interview

It would be a betrayal of the therapeutic relationship to talk with a third party about a patient without their knowledge. The clinician has to get the patient's permission first, and this should be documented. In family interviews, the distinction between gathering and giving information is not entirely clear cut, and this demands clarity as to whether there are matters that the patient does not want disclosed. There are legal and ethical obligations on any doctor in these situations. Conversely, however, where the patient is happy for information to be given, there is no excuse for withholding it from the family.

There are some complexities with regard to the patient's consent. Firstly, in the UK, under certain circumstances, there is a legal obligation to consult with relatives prior to legally detaining the patient. Secondly, where there is a significant element of risk, or in order to assess someone who is seriously unwell, it may be necessary to override their explicit wishes and take information from informants. Thirdly, where a third party is at risk, it may be necessary to break confidentiality. This is a legal obligation if a child is at risk, but it may involve warning an adult where, for example, there are jealous delusions. These breaches of professional boundaries should not be taken lightly, and must be capable of justification to the patient. Where breaches of boundaries occur, reasons for this should be documented, and the patient should be told about it as soon as is practicably possible.

If you are interviewing more than one person, it is best to have two interviewers in the room. Family interviews are potentially complicated situations, and it is difficult to both conduct the interview and observe what is going on. Naturally enough, the considerations set out in Chapter 12 apply. It is particularly

> **BOX 13.1 Families are systems**
>
> Families can be thought of as small social systems. The membership of a family alters only slowly and families tend to follow stable rules of interaction. However, families face many threats to their stability and integrity. Family members die. Children grow up and adults grow old, which changes the way they behave. Conflict occurs from time to time, or it may be continuous. Families have to cope with children leaving home. These are internal and intrinsic sources of family instability. There are also external threats, for example, disease, unemployment or infidelity.
>
> In order to prevent the family disintegrating in response to these threats, families have homeostatic mechanisms to resist change, and adaptive mechanisms to incorporate change when it cannot be resisted. A system cannot maintain a stable configuration without such mechanisms. The family would break up as soon as it faces any serious problem if it does not have them. When threats arise, the family as a system tries to find an adaptation that involves minimal change. For example, the loss of the parenting role when one's children marry is often replaced with a similar, though attenuated, parenting role towards grandchildren. Maintaining the stability of a family is a high priority for its members.
>
> During the process of finding a partner, settling down and forming a new family, there are powerful forces that drive people to reproduce patterns of interaction which are familiar from their family of origin. These patterns are comfortable. We tend to choose partners who are like ourselves and who come from similar families. Most people, when dealing with their children, have the disturbing experience of acting and speaking just like their own parents, despite trying to avoid this. One can rarely create new patterns of family behaviour through an act of will.
>
> Interactions within families follow idiosyncratic and unspoken rules. They are often based upon family myths, which include shared beliefs about the family. For example, a family myth might be that expressing overt anger is extremely destructive. This might lead to a rule that anger must not be verbalised, which avoids destructive arguments. An adverse consequence might be that anger is expressed by protracted sullen silences and therefore conflict resolution is difficult.
>
> Individuals can come to play special roles within families. For example, troublesome children who are hard to discipline can become the scapegoat for everything that goes wrong within the family ('Your mother and I are separating because of you'). The academically successful can come to carry the whole family's aspirations for self-improvement. They may then find it difficult to lower their personal ambitions when the need arises.
>
> When it is hard to understand why families are behaving as they are, it can be useful to consider whether these kinds of factors may be shaping their behaviour.

important for the team members to be clear as to their agenda, the length of the interview and who is going to lead it.

In general, patients should be included in family interviews, even where this is awkward. Openness is always the best governing principle, even when it makes things difficult in the short run. Taking the line of least resistance, on the other hand, often leads you to a much more difficult and dishonest position in the long run. Nonetheless the problems of including the patient in the interview are very real. Patients who are actively unwell, especially those who are manic or suffering from schizophreniform psychosis, can find family interviews stressful. They may become more disturbed during the interview as a consequence. Family members can find some information very difficult to give in the presence of the patient, including simply stating that they think they are mentally unwell. Generally speaking, patients should only be excluded if this is their own wish or if there is a real risk of tangible harm occurring if they are included. Certainly, the psychiatrist should never say anything to a family that he would not be happy to say to the patient himself.

At the start of the interview

Following the usual principles, introductions are important. Families and friends are often very unfamiliar with professional roles, and saying 'I'm the SHO' or 'I'm an OT' may convey nothing at all to them. 'I'm the doctor based on the ward' or 'I'm an occupational therapist and I work with people on their daily living skills' is much more meaningful. The family must be told how long the interview will last, but they should always be told that there will be further opportunities to meet. 'One-off' interviewing creates an intolerable pressure on a family to deal with everything that matters to them within the interview.

Introductions need to be made in both directions. It is essential to know who everyone is, and the nature of their relationship with the patient. Sometimes, family members bring their friends to support them; the friend has a relationship with the patient's relative but not with the patient. You need to know this.

At this stage, before the discussion has started, you have to state that there are limitations to what you can disclose. Families have longstanding and deep relationships with the patient, and, understandably enough, they rarely see why the rules of confidentiality should apply to them. However, patients often want confidences kept from those closest to them. Acknowledging that something is being withheld creates a partial disclosure. Consequently, confidentiality has to be raised as a principle, rather than waiting until you cannot answer a question (thus revealing where a secret lies).

Having completed these preliminaries, it is often useful to set out an explicit agenda for the meeting. This involves clearly stating what you hope to achieve in the course of the interview, and inviting the family to do likewise. Where they do not have a clear agenda, this may involve asking each of them how they see the patient's problem. Indeed, it is useful to ask this in any case, as the question often exposes misunderstandings, undisclosed items of history and a range of other useful information.

If there seems to be an unrealistically huge joint agenda, the family can be asked to prioritise the two or three matters that are most important to them. Other agenda items can be dealt with at a later meeting.

During the interview

Controlling family interviews

If you have prepared the ground properly, the majority of routine family interviews are straightforward. They are not generally difficult to control. There is often a family spokesman, who does most of the talking. From time to time, it is helpful to invite other family members to say what they think, or to ask whether they agree. This ensures that all views can be aired. It can also help unlock the discussion, should it start going in circles.

All psychiatrists will occasionally have difficult interviews with families, and the experience can be quite aversive. Families sometimes come feeling defensive, aggrieved or guilty. They may be angry with the psychiatrist, with the patient or with each other. This can make it difficult to have a fruitful interview. The presence of a number of angry people in the room can be very uncomfortable, and though it is very uncommon for real aggression to emerge, it is not helpful to continue if emotions are running out of control. It is important to recognise when an interview has become counterproductive and to close it.

There are two techniques that can be helpful in disarming conflict in family interviews. These are positive connotation and acknowledgement of fallibility.

Positive connotation is a family therapy technique. It means that the behaviour of family members is acknowledged by the doctor as being well-intentioned. This stance is maintained even with regard to behaviour that the psychiatrist feels is misguided or counterproductive. Behaviour is not directly criticised, but is construed as the consequence of family members attempting to do their best under difficult circumstances. This has the advantage of usually being true. Even when it is not strictly true, it can free defensive family members from feeling attacked. It is intended to place the clinician outside of the family dynamic, as he endorses everyone equally.

Acknowledgement of fallibility is an interpersonal strategy that runs counter to medical culture. It seems self-evident that one should admit mistakes and apologise for them. Explanations and apologies tend to avoid severe problems in relationships and, ultimately, litigation. Unfortunately, doctors have to work at this. However, acknowledgement of fallibility involves more than simply putting your hands up to genuine errors. It also involves expressing regret over (or apologising for) incidents and factors that are outside of your control. For example, in the face of serious mental illness, families' distress can focus on relative minutiae. Consequently, families may have grievances that seem 'unreasonable'. In a high-risk situation leading to compulsory admission, they may complain about the involvement of the police. They may protest because a previously highly aggressive patient now seems rather drugged. It is usually helpful to acknowledge that such matters are very distressing and to apologise for them, even though they are an inevitable, or even appropriate part of the treatment process. This is not to say you can disown such aspects of care. You certainly should never imply that someone else's conscientious actions were inappropriate. The recognition that the treatment is imperfect and that you are fallible is both true and disarming in many circumstances. The ability to strike this position requires professional self-confidence, and is not possible if you feel significant defensiveness over what has happened.

Obtaining information from families

Family interviews are unusual settings. Answers to questions can be corrected or debated by family members. Compared with individual interviewing, a family interview often provides a clearer and richer picture of how things have developed. A clinical hypothesis can be tested by putting it to the family and asking them what they think. However, in gathering information, it is helpful to focus on events and specific behaviours. Families will often talk about feelings and causational theories. This is natural enough, but the psychiatrist needs to know what has actually happened and specific examples of behaviour, so that the context and the sequence of events can be fully explored.

Sometimes you want to know about patterns of behaviour within families. This can be helpful in assessing, for example, the degree to which the patient is exposed to high expressed emotion responses. It is usually best to ask a third person within the family about the interaction between two family members. The third person is likely to have a clearer view of the interaction, and is more likely to be able to describe it without re-enacting the emotions. For example, a sibling can be asked about a parent's responses to the patient. The two participants are more likely to tell you how the other makes them feel than what they actually do. In any case, they may not be aware of their own habitual patterns of response. The process of asking one family member about the interactions between two other family members can be repeated with respect to each dyad in turn. This even-handed process can reveal a great deal about the way a family functions. In systemic family therapy, this is called circular questioning.

BOX 13.2 'Don't tell her we told you, but she's planning to kill Gran'

Caroline is a 20-year-old student. Her family have noticed that for over a year or so she has become increasingly suspicious and irritable. Eventually, she takes a serious overdose. On assessment, she is found to be suffering from schizophrenia, and she agrees to be admitted to hospital. Several days later, her mother phones the ward doctor, Dr Smith. She is very worried, and wants to tell Dr Smith something in strict confidence. She has been reading her daughter's diary. Caroline has written several entries to the effect that her grandmother has been replaced by a demon and that she must be killed in order to restore her true grandmother. There was a kitchen knife with the diary. The old lady is disabled by heart disease and lives in the household.

Caroline's mother is extremely concerned about the welfare of both her daughter and her own mother. However, she does not want to do anything to jeopardise her relationship with Caroline, as she realises that Caroline is going to need her family's support over the next few years. She does not want their daughter to know that she has been through her possessions. She does not want Caroline to feel that she thinks she is a potential murderer. If Dr Smith mentions the contents of the diary, Caroline will know that the information could only have come from her mother. She does not want the diary to be directly mentioned. Naively, she believes that the knowledge that the entries exist will allow the psychiatrist to assess and contain her daughter's dangerousness.

Dr Smith is in a difficult position. Caroline's mother has good reasons for secrecy, albeit based on some misconceptions about the powers of psychiatrists. However, she can only explore the information by confronting Caroline with the contents of the diary, in breach of her undertaking of confidentiality to her mother.

Sometimes, it is possible to infer aspects of family functioning from behaviour in the interview. For example, patterns of dependency and hostility may be revealed in the choice of seating positions, and responses to distress say something about the quality of relationships. Family beliefs, myths and rules may be implied during the interview. However, it is important to bear in mind that these are always inferences, which should normally be tested by asking the family about the accuracy of the observation.

There is a very common problem that arises in family interviews, and that is the conditional disclosure of information. An example is set out in Box 13.2.

It can be hard to understand why families want to conceal the fact that they have made a disclosure. The risk of an argument or of unpleasantness often seems trivial in the face of the importance of the information disclosed. However, there are all kinds of barriers to frankness within families, and there is often more at stake than is immediately obvious.

When a family member is mentally unwell, relationships can feel very fragile. Disclosure of secrets carries a higher than usual risk of breakdown of relationships and therefore threatens the integrity of the family. Disclosures may involve breaking family rules (for example, 'we don't involve outsiders in our problems'). Families have sometimes colluded with the patient, for example by agreeing with them that delusions are true. Having avoided conflict in this way, a disclosure risks revealing that the collusion was dishonest and that they have been effectively lying for weeks or months.

Although families request undertakings of confidentiality for reasons that are salient, wherever possible you should decline to make an undertaking to conceal a disclosure. There are two good reasons for this. Firstly, families often suppose that once the psychiatrist knows the information, he has some power to get the patient to tell him about it. In fact, it is almost always impossible to do anything with the information unless you can confront the patient with it. Secondly, concealment introduces dishonesty between the psychiatrist and the patient, and this often causes problems later, for example, when the information appears in a report. If these reasons are explained most families will understand, and will withdraw the demand for confidentiality of disclosure. Dealing with the problems caused by disclosure becomes a joint task for family and professionals. However, some families remain very perturbed. Occasionally, as there is no duty of confidentiality to the family, you have to go ahead and tell the patient anyway. Even if it is possible to observe the family's wishes without adverse consequences, you can never make an unconditional undertaking to withhold information from a patient. There is always a possibility that circumstances will arise where you have to tell.

Giving information to families

In giving information to families, it is particularly easy to make an assumption about what they already know and hence break confidentiality. You cannot assume that all family members know what you know, and even apparently innocuous information can be very sensitive in some families. You should only give information when you are clear about the family members' understanding of the situation, knowing what information is common currency and what is not. It is important to go slowly, with lots of repetition.

At the end of the interview

At the end of the interview, there is an opportunity to give any message that you particularly want the family to hear, which will usually be a reiteration of something you have said earlier. One should not underestimate how easily messages can be misinterpreted in these interviews, no matter how intelligent the participants may be. Consequently, important messages need to be stated very clearly and simply. It can be helpful to invite the family to make any closing observations or remarks; families will often come up with novel solutions to problems if given the opportunity. Generally speaking, it is helpful to invite the family to meet with you again if they want to, and to state that they may forget what you have said and that you do not mind going over it again at a later date.

Finally, team members need to debrief and reflect on the interview, in order to share observations and to make a record of the interview. If a new hypothesis about the patient or the family emerges, this needs to be recorded, together with a record of the evidence supporting it. The record should state clearly what information the family have been given and any undertakings that have been made to them, for example with respect to future meetings or to avoid certain treatments. When relationships with families go wrong, it is invaluable to have a contemporaneous record of what was said to them. This can help to rescue the relationship.

The accompanied patient

Patients sometimes arrive at interviews unexpectedly accompanied by a family member or friend. This is usually an attempt to support an anxious patient, though sometimes the family member also wants to influence the interview. Occasionally, the family member is an unwelcome intruder into the interview. The interviewer must have some time alone with the patient, either at the beginning or the end of the interview. Without this, it is impossible to know how the patient feels about the relative's presence, and there is a risk that the interview can be very misleading.

It is reasonable to ask to see the patient alone to begin with. A clear statement at the beginning that the relative will be invited in later will usually avoid attempts to force a joint interview. Very anxious patients may resist this, in which case the pair can be seen together at the outset. Towards the end, when the patient is likely to have relaxed, you can ask the relative to leave for the final part of the interview. What you must avoid is the situation where the patient is never seen alone. In our experience, this nearly always leads to the relative's agenda overwhelming and submerging the patient's concerns.

Children and carers

Mental illnesses do not just happen in people's minds, they happen in their lives. Severe and enduring mental illnesses have a major impact on families. It is well recognised that those who care for the mentally ill, usually family members, experience high levels of stress and are vulnerable to becoming depressed themselves. They can become very isolated. They need information, support and a life of their own. When carers do become depressed, this can have an adverse impact upon the patient's mental health, setting up a vicious circle of stress and mental illness.

It is important that mental health professionals should be attentive to carer's needs. Families mostly provide care without question and they tend not to express their needs. Mental health professionals need to have a high awareness that carers may be struggling. The patient's needs and the carer's needs may be in conflict, and so when a carer is assessed in their own right, this should be dealt with by a different team (or where this is impossible, a different team member), and independently of the assessment of the patient's needs. Since the Carers Recognition and Services Act 1995, carers in the UK have a right to an independent assessment of their needs, and their rights have been strengthened by several subsequent Acts of Parliament.

Not all families are benign or well-intentioned, and they may, for example, use the patient as a cash cow through the benefit system. Malignant families create real dilemmas for clinical teams, as it can be hard to curtail their activities and to get them out of the patient's life. When it is impossible to work with a family, it is nearly always necessary to involve social workers and to use legislation designed to protect vulnerable adults.

Child protection procedures exist to prevent children from coming to serious harm. In the UK, there is a legal obligation to place the needs of children over the needs of adults. Child protection is a formal and overriding responsibility of all health professionals, even where the child at risk is unknown to the professional, or where the risk is to children in general. There are no ethical or legal exceptions.

It is always important to have a low threshold for initiating formal assessment of a patient's child. This often means serious disruption to the therapeutic relationship with the patient, but it cannot be avoided. If you have a high threshold for referral, then some children will come to harm when this could be avoided. This is not to say that mentally ill parents necessarily represent a risk to their children or are poor parents. In the course of a career, however, all psychiatrists will come across some patients who are both.

The impact of parental mental illness on children is far more far-reaching than the kinds of problems that require action under child protection procedures. When the patient has dependent children, the adverse effects of mental illness and of psychiatric treatments are amplified. Mentally ill parents sometimes do things that frighten their children. Suicide attempts leave children feeling insecure. Sedative side effects of medication and preoccupation with psychiatric symptoms make it difficult to function as a parent, and the children lose important parental attention. Often, the other parent is distracted and unavailable to the children. These problems can be quite protracted, and they occur whilst the child's development presses on regardless. Consequently, the effects can be persistent.

British culture has a strong tendency to try to protect children from unhappiness through denial. For example, children are frequently excluded from unhappy family events, such as funerals. In a similar spirit, families often pretend to children that mental illness and hospitalisation are not happening, or that they are insignificant. The adults are often frightened by mental illness, and do not understand it. This makes it difficult to offer the children an explanation, and it is easier to avoid the subject. In fact, even young children are usually very aware of parental illness.

Community mental health teams have a high awareness of the needs of their patients' children, and have a role in ensuring that practical steps are taken to avoid emotional harm to them. This is far below the threshold that invokes child protection procedures. Low key interventions are far from 100% protective, but they achieve a great deal more than doing nothing at all. Children need, above all, help to understand what has happened. They do not necessarily need specialist help. Children can and should be included in family interviews. Someone in the team has to take the trouble to explain to the family how they can tell the children what has happened in terms that they can understand. If the family cannot do this, a team member may have to do it for them. Once it is recognised that the children's needs should be attended to, the interventions are relatively simple.

Long-term relationships with families

Just as therapeutic relationships can last for decades, so too can relationships with patients' families. The vast majority of these relationships are helpful and of good quality. Occasionally, the relationship with the family is better than the relationship with the patient. The professionals and the family start to routinely conspire to manipulate the patient. Tempting though this can be, it is a betrayal of the relationship with the patient, which then can never be improved, even if a new team takes over.

Occasionally, families turn out to have attitudes towards the patient or his illness that are overindulgent, neglectful or bizarre. It is very tempting to avoid confronting these attitudes in the interests of sustaining the relationship with the family. However, this is usually a mistake. If you do not tackle such problems at the beginning of the relationship with the family, it is generally impossible to do anything about it later. Confrontation need not be aggressive, but there should be a clear statement of disagreement. For example, if a family believes that individual psychoanalysis is the treatment of choice for their daughter's schizophrenia, going along with the idea on the basis that there is a long waiting list will tend to create a difficulty when the daughter comes to the top of the waiting list. An early statement of disagreement may be awkward, but it serves the patient's interests much better in the long run.

Finally, you have to bear in mind that families are systems that can only be imperfectly understood. When a professional gives information to a family, it can have an unexpected impact. It may alter perceptions as to the nature and causes of the patient's problems. This can, in turn, significantly alter interactions within the family. Altered interactions can be helpful, but they can also destabilise families. Marriages that have survived years of difficult behaviour may abruptly break down if a psychiatrist changes the family's view of the patient's responsibility for their own actions. There is little that you can do to prevent this, but one has to anticipate that dramatic responses to family interviews will sometimes happen.

Main points in this chapter

1. Families, even dysfunctional ones, are important to patients, and you have to be able to work with them.
2. Families are systems with homeostatic mechanisms. This may explain some aspects of family behaviour.
3. Family interviews require the patient's consent. The patient should participate.
4. It is easy to accidentally breach confidentiality in family interviews.
5. A handful of special techniques, such as circular questioning, positive connotation and acknowledgement of fallibility, make difficult interviews a lot easier.
6. Disclosure of information should not be accepted on a conditional basis.
7. Patient's families, especially their dependent children, have important needs. A small amount of attention to these can make a big difference.
8. Recovery from mental illness is more likely where there is a three-way alliance between family, patient and professionals.

14

In the community

Why bother to interview patients at home?

Psychiatry developed within large institutions, and the clinical practice of psychiatry still bears a clear imprint of its institutional origins. In the UK, the majority of the big mental hospitals have closed, but the patterns of working established there continue in many of the new, smaller, more dispersed facilities. A proportion of the profession is nostalgic for a more genteel working life in the asylums. There are pressure groups that campaign for a return to more institutional, and custodial, forms of care.

This attachment to the past seems to us to be extraordinary, as the evidence for the superiority of community psychiatry over institutional psychiatry is overwhelming. Institutional psychiatry is disliked by patients and causes secondary handicap. Asylum staff were well-intentioned, and the asylums were the best form of care available at the time. However, the institutions were barren neglectful places to live, and many chronically unwell patients experienced empty and wasted lives, their symptoms worsened by the environment that was supposed to be helping them to recover.

The perception that community psychiatry is associated with an increased risk to patients and the public has no basis in empirical evidence. In our opinion, the perception has probably arisen because, with the closure of asylums, adverse incidents that once passed unnoticed behind institutional walls now occur in public view. Our attachment to community psychiatry may be based on our personal dislike of hospitals, but it has strong support from the evidence base and from humanitarian considerations.

In the twenty-first century, British psychiatry is in an odd state of development. For the most part, we have physically left the asylums, but we have not yet fully arrived in the community either. The problem is this: in order to practice community psychiatry, the psychiatrist has to leave his office. This cannot be done by proxy. The fact that the psychiatrist works with other staff who visit the patient at home is insufficient to secure the advantages of community practice.

The whole team has to work within the community it serves. Community psychiatry involves assessing and treating patients in their own environments, primarily within their own homes. This does not just avoid the damaging effects of institutional psychiatry, it also brings changes in perspective and an alteration in power relationships. Everything about the practice of psychiatry is changed by taking the psychiatrist to the patient rather than vice versa.

The process of conducting an interview with a patient at home is not significantly different from a clinical interview. It does require a good understanding of both multi-disciplinary and family interviewing, but the actual skills deployed are much the same, irrespective of the location. However, within the patient's home there is a very different type of information available regarding their habits, tastes, routines, lifestyle and social environment. We all create our home environments, which come to reflect profound personal characteristics. No matter how long you talk to the patient and informants in an office, a mass of qualitative information is lost, which can only be accessed by actually going to the patient's home.

In order to utilise this rich source of information, it has to be noticed. Some people notice things more easily than others, but it is also a skill that can be developed. Noticing involves an active curiosity, and has to be linked to a willingness to ask 'why?' Noticing includes, for example, both understanding that personal collections of books reveal important patterns of interests and knowing that a construction of an empty plastic bottle, silver foil and drinking straws is a bong (or crack pipe). There is information evident in a patient's home that can save time by providing answers to standard history-taking questions. However, the real advantage is in the new types of information that are available, and in the powerful, accurate and enduring snapshot that one obtains of the patient's life.

The other big advantage of community interviewing over office interviewing is that there is a major, though complicated, difference in the relationship between the psychiatrist and the patient from the outset. Psychiatrists sometimes have to exert control over patients, and are frequently involved in trying to persuade them to do things that they do not want to do. However, the overarching long-term task is to get alongside the patient, to work together towards the restoration of independence and autonomy. Control is most easily achieved in the psychiatrist's environment, but it is a short-term objective. Getting alongside patients is more easily achieved in the patient's environment.

There is nothing particularly strange or surprising about this. To take a simple example, psychiatrists often run late. There is a significant difference between the patient being kept waiting for half an hour in an unfamiliar waiting room full of strangers and being kept waiting for half an hour in their own home. The former is stressful and aversive. The latter is, at worst, a minor inconvenience.

Inviting someone into your home means that the interview is proceeding on your territory and, psychologically, on your terms. Many patients who would never agree to actively going to see a psychiatrist in his office will allow you to visit at home. There is a major difference between allowing a psychiatrist to visit to see if he can help, and making the more positive decision that you need to see a psychiatrist and then taking the trouble to go and see him. People usually come to your house to offer you a service. In contrast, a visit to a hospital or to a doctor's surgery places the patient in a more subservient and supplicant position.

So, the simple change of location changes the relationship, such that it is easier to form a cooperative partnership with the patient as opposed to a relationship where the psychiatrist tries to get the patient to bend to his will. One reason for trying to get alongside patients, rather than dominating them, is that it works better. People, generally speaking, do not like being told what to do. They are much more likely to follow an agreed plan that they have helped to formulate with the psychiatrist.

The better information and the different type of relationship that come with community interviewing allows a team to deal with emergencies differently and to avoid inpatient admissions. It is far easier to treat someone who is psychotic at home if you have seen the home and met family and friends. Risk assessment is more accurate, and plans can be agreed and implemented immediately. Inpatient admission is the part of psychiatric treatment which is most disliked by patients, and it is far easier to avoid it if the psychiatrist and the rest of the team see the patient at home.

Some types of psychiatric problems can only be properly assessed in the patient's home. For example, the day-to-day functioning of patients suffering from dementia is not necessarily closely correlated with the objective cognitive deficit. It is their ability to cope at home which forms the most important part of the assessment. There can be a significant difference between the patient's general orientation and their orientation in their home environment. Routine tasks, such as preparation of food, can be witnessed and critical safety issues, such as the patient's ability to operate gas appliances, can be tested. A clinic assessment might accurately reveal the degree of objective cognitive impairment, but it is very difficult to accurately assess functional ability in that setting. People with cognitive impairment tend to function at their worst in hospitals, which is why old-age psychiatrists were amongst the pioneers of home assessment.

There are many further advantages to working in the community, but it must be acknowledged that there are also some significant problems.

Confidentiality

Confidentiality faces some novel threats when working in the community, and it is easy to get caught out. For example, it is easiest to arrange a visit through a telephone call, which is no problem if the patient lives alone. However, if you call and a different family member answers, you may immediately breach confidentiality by giving an honest response to the reasonable question 'Who is calling?' Some such traps can be avoided (for example, by writing to the patient and inviting them to call you to arrange an appointment), but some cannot. For example, because of the strong relationship between deprivation and serious mental disorder, in any community psychiatrist's patch, there is likely to be a concentration of patients in certain locations. After a short while in the job, all anonymity is lost, and you are quite likely to be spotted and identified whilst waiting at someone's doorstep. Even if you are not personally identified, within an inner city community an unknown man in a suit is likely to be spotted and taken to be a policeman or a bailiff. There are likely to be questions about your identity.

Intrusiveness

Most patients prefer to be seen at home, but a few prefer office interviews. One reason is exactly the type of breach of confidentiality set out above. However, a variety of other factors, such as previous experience of involuntary admission, shame over neglected accommodation and the presence of domineering relatives, can mean that the patient finds the prospect of a home visit intrusive. For this reason, patients have to have the option of an office visit if this is their preference, though under these circumstances it is always important to try to understand what is driving their reluctance to be seen at home. It is likely that the reasons will be important in understanding the patient, and it is often possible to reassure them sufficiently to allow a later home visit.

Lack of control of the environment

The main problem with lack of control over the environment is that it means you do not have full control of the interview. Other family members may unexpectedly be present, and it can be difficult to get them out of the room (it is their home, after all). Even if they agree to leave the room, they may be able to overhear the interview, which can be inhibiting for the patient and the interviewer alike. It can often mean that an assessment is only partially completed. Although there is usually an opportunity to complete the process at a later time, this complicates basic information gathering. There is no doubt that it is better to get the task completed in a single session, not least because the patient is likely to be anxious to hear your opinion. However, in the community, assessment often has to be carried out in phases. This requires clarity about what you have omitted and what you do not know, both of which should be clearly recorded in the notes.

However, under many circumstances, the unexpected presence of other family members can be opportunistically exploited, for example, in order to get an informant history. It is usually better to utilise the opportunities present in the situation as you find it, rather than ploughing on with your original agenda under circumstances that make it difficult to achieve. Conversely, the presence of small children is much less problematic in the patient's own home than in a clinic setting, as they are far less disruptive at home, and can often be safely left in a different room.

Interruptions, especially the arrival of unexpected visitors, are a real problem in the community, and there is not much that can be done about it. Patients mostly sort these problems out for you, though some visitors will bowl in and want to know who you are, posing problems over confidentiality. One has to be prepared to improvise in these situations, and sometimes to abandon the interview altogether, to return at a later time.

Professional boundaries

Maintaining boundaries is more difficult in the community. The psychiatrist's office offers an actual and a symbolic formality, which emphasises the different positions of the doctor and the patient. Roles are more ambiguous in the home. Most patients offer you a cup of tea or coffee when you arrive, and participation in these ordinary social rituals is part of the process that makes for a different relationship. However, the offer (or, more importantly, the acceptance) of an alcoholic beverage clearly breaks a boundary. More subtly, it is easy for the relationship to shift towards something inappropriately reciprocal. Although one has to behave in a more informal way in the community, this demands a constant awareness of professional boundaries.

Some patients, of course, tend to threaten boundaries because of the nature of their problem, for example, some patients with borderline personality disorder who crave intimacy. Some types of patients cannot be visited at home appropriately by some types of professionals, for example, male patients with a history of sexual aggression are usually best not seen at home alone by female staff. These situations are another reason why there is always a need for residual clinic interviewing: there are no one-size-fits-all approaches in clinical psychiatry.

Inefficiency

Few psychiatrists seem to doubt the superiority of home visits over clinic appointments, but some (perhaps the more institutionalised) object that it is impractical to abandon clinics because home visiting is 'inefficient'. They point out that they see a patient every 15 min in clinic, and that it is impossible to maintain this work rate if you add travelling time. On top of this, interviewing at home demands flexibility, as a second, or indeed third, visit may be needed to complete an assessment, whereas assessment can almost always be completed in a single one-hour appointment in the clinic.

What this fails to take into account is the alteration to team working and to the whole face of clinical practice that occurs when you move into the community. Where more than one team member is involved with a patient, follow-up visits can be conducted jointly, which saves time on meetings. Because it is easier to delay or cancel home visits than outpatient appointments, working practices are intrinsically more flexible. The better quality of home interviews means that they can occur less frequently. Letters can be dictated in the car between visits, which allows both team members to influence the content. Psychiatric clinics have very high non-attendance rates, whereas the rate of failed home visits is far lower. This makes the use of time more efficient. Routine appointments can be reduced to periodic multidisciplinary reviews of treatment, often only once a year. Clinics, on the other hand, tend to have an autonomous rebooking cycle, which demands more frequent visits.

Some institutionalised psychiatrists concede that this style of practice is practical in cities, but object that it is impractical in rural settings where the population is more dispersed. In fact, in rural settings the majority of the population tend to live together in settlements, and only a minority are very dispersed. It might be that one cannot offer a true community service to very dispersed rural areas, but it is still possible to offer it to their neighbours in small towns and large villages.

Even if the objection that community psychiatry is prohibitively time-consuming were true, it would not change the strongest argument for this style of working, which is that it works better, and is generally preferred by patients.

Dogs

Issues of safety are dealt with in Chapter 16, but no discussion of home interviewing would be complete without mentioning dogs. Unfortunately, the British are a nation of dog lovers, but dogs are not, in general, a species of psychiatrist lovers (though some dogs have an erotic interest in psychiatrists' legs). Ethology tells us that whilst dogs come in a wide variety of sizes, they are all territorial pack animals with a strong sense of hierarchy and conspicuous dentition. Dogs are a significant distraction in the clinical situation. Even when calm, certain breeds of dog, such as bull terriers, can present a surprisingly intimidating facial expression. Large dogs are not necessarily the biggest problem. Small dogs can be very aggressive, and are a particular problem for those of us who have lost line-of-sight contact with our shoes. Being bitten is not the only risk. Stepping on a pet is a poor prelude to a sensitive interview.

The point about dogs is that you need to know about them. It is worth asking about the presence of dogs within the household prior to visiting. Dog owners are rarely aware of the effect of their pet on visitors, and it is usually necessary to ask for them to be removed from the interview. It is sensible to have a method for flagging the clinical notes for the presence of dogs.

Psychiatric emergencies in the community

The concept of a psychiatric emergency is difficult, because mental illnesses tend to evolve relatively slowly, and quite often it is not the patient who thinks that there is an emergency. Certainly, the old adage that, in psychiatry, the term 'emergency' merely indicates that someone (patient, family member or professional) is frightened is true, and it is also true that emergencies often relate to factors other than changes in the patient's mental state. For example, 'emergencies' often arise on a Friday afternoon or before bank holidays, because there is an anxiety that something bad will happen, not immediately, but before the next time help is readily available. Alternatively, emergencies can arise when the patient's mental state has shown little change, but someone else has suddenly become aware that they are unwell.

The essential components in resolving psychiatric emergencies in all settings are:

- to try to understand how the patient is experiencing the situation.
- to be clear who is in charge.
- to respond to the objective risks, not to speculative fears.
- to keep everybody's anxiety under control (including your own).
- to take the time that is needed to resolve the situation, rather than acting under external time pressure (e.g. because a shift is ending). This often means retreating and taking time to think.

The good thing about attending an emergency situation in the community is that you can see for yourself what is happening, and you can gain a clear understanding of how the situation has developed. It may be possible to negotiate a treatment plan with the patient because you will be involved in delivering it, and this can be helpful in avoiding compulsory admission. However, even if the patient was not frightened to begin with, he is likely to become so as an emergency assessment proceeds. Fear, almost always, makes people's mental state deteriorate. The assessing psychiatrist is often intruding into the patient's home and this can understandably make people very angry. You have little control over the environment. There may well be frightened or distressed family members present. There may be ambulance staff, police officers, social workers, general practitioners and emergency vehicles. None of this will calm the patient down. At best, he will think he is likely to be admitted to hospital against his will. He is quite likely to put a more paranoid interpretation on the situation. What he certainly will not do is fail to notice the developing situation.

Planning is generally important, and this means collating as much information as possible before visiting the patient. When things go wrong during emergencies in the community, it can be distressing to later learn that an identical sequence of events occurred a few months earlier. Consequently, if it is possible, prior to visiting you should speak to someone who knows the patient.

Often, it is best to have a low key initial visit before involving other services, though this is not always safe. Once you are in contact with the patient, it is a good principle to tell them what you intend to do at each stage. There is no role for misleading the patient or 'jumping' them, except under the most dangerous circumstances. Many patients, equipped with knowledge of your plans, will decide to go along with them.

Generally speaking, one's overall approach needs to be heavily modified in emergency circumstances. There is little point in attempting to do a comprehensive assessment, as it is likely to be impossible and, in any case, background histories taken under such circumstances tend to be misleading. These are dynamic, evolving situations, and it is the decision-making process that is most important. You often have to make decisions without comprehensive information, on the basis of the balance of factors as the assessment proceeds. It is important to recognise that your decisions may prove to be less than optimal once full information is available. The strength of your conclusions needs to reflect the available evidence.

Some emergency interviews happen in public or semi-public places; crowds can form, and strangers or neighbours can intervene. Some interviews are extremely fragmentary and are conducted, for example, whilst pursuing the patient through a busy shopping precinct. It can be difficult to maintain a proper professional persona, patient confidentiality and the personal dignity and safety of all involved. You have to be prepared to give up once it is obvious that the assessment cannot be brought to a satisfactory conclusion.

Main points in this chapter

1. Community psychiatry involves working within the community rather than the clinic.
2. Interviewing patients in their own home involves no new techniques, but does offer a new type of clinical information.
3. Working with patients in their own environment changes the therapeutic relationship and the nature of multidisciplinary working.
4. There are some difficulties in community interviewing, especially concerning confidentiality and maintenance of boundaries.
5. Psychiatric emergencies in the community are not easy to manage, but they benefit from planning and an awareness of the patient's point of view.

Part VI

Drawing it all together

Assessment does not just involve systematic collection of information and careful observation. There is eventually a need to bring information together and to make critical evaluations. One such evaluation involves arriving at a diagnosis. As discussed in Chapter 1, this is relatively straightforward, thanks to modern operationalised diagnostic systems, but it is in itself an inadequate way of understanding the patient. There are three other evaluation tasks that are important in every case, namely the assessment of personality, the assessment of risk and the communication of one's findings to others. Assessment of personality and risk are complicated by some intrinsic ambiguities. The communication of findings is a difficult task which is given scant attention in training. No one can be expected to learn how to do it well without properly understanding the task.

15

Personality

Personality is an intuitively simple construct which is well understood by most people, so it is perhaps surprising that theoretical and practical issues concerning personality are amongst the most difficult in psychiatry. Personality is important. It is impossible to practice psychiatry satisfactorily without a good understanding of personality. Empathic understanding of others depends upon an appreciation of the different types of personalities, and of the range of ways in which people experience the world as a consequence. No one can make a credible diagnosis of personality disorder unless they understand normal personality.

Personality is more than just the backdrop against which mental disorder plays. Personality profoundly shapes symptoms and behaviour. It creates those personal vulnerabilities that contribute to mental disorder and the personal strengths that help people to find a way back to good health.

Understanding the patient's main personality characteristics is an essential part of every psychiatric assessment. This is made difficult by three factors:

- Psychiatry has no generally accepted model of personality. There is a theoretical muddle and consequently outsiders often find psychiatrists' attitude to personality problems hard to understand. Models of personality functioning are discussed in Box 15.1.
- Very few people can accurately describe themselves as they are experienced by others. The assessment of personality, therefore, depends on a degree of inference and, in cases where personality issues are significant, access to more than one account.
- The diagnosis of personality disorder has a pejorative implication that has survived repeated application of euphemisms. The whole diagnostic group can be misused to pass a value judgement upon a patient or to diagnose unpopular patients out of the service. Whilst the concept remains useful, the tendency for 'personality disorder' to imply 'unworthy' creates difficulties with respect to objectivity.

Personality is that range of characteristic behavioural responses that a person deploys to cope with the world and their feelings. The greater the range and variety of responses within this behavioural repertoire, the more likely it is that

BOX 15.1 Models of personality

The various ways of thinking about personality and personality disorder can be broadly divided into three types of models: trait, categorical and structural. They are not necessarily mutually exclusive, and there are strengths and weaknesses in each.

Trait models

In these models, behavioural characteristics are seen to group together as traits, each of which exists on a continuous spectrum. An example would be the tendency to show anxious responses. Some people only react anxiously under serious threat, whilst others show it on minimal provocation. The majority of people are distributed on an axis between these extremes. An individual's personality is the consequence of the combination of different traits displayed to different degrees. Normal personalities are those where each trait is present near the population mean. Abnormal personalities have one or more traits at the extreme.

Personality traits can be measured reliably using standardised instruments. There is a plausible link with behavioural genetics; it is possible to breed aggressive dogs or anxious mice, and family studies in humans suggest that behavioural traits are at least partly inherited.

There are some weaknesses with this type of model. It is unclear whether personality traits exist as independent behavioural variables or whether they are artefacts of psychometric tests. Traits can be broken down into smaller, more numerous components or brought together to construct fewer, larger variables. Different individuals with similar psychometric personality profiles can be quite different, suggesting that these theories are missing something. Personality develops and changes throughout life, but trait theories cannot easily incorporate developmental factors.

Categorical models

These suggest that personality characteristics cluster together, creating distinctive types, for example the overdriven, tense, time-aware type A personality which is associated with cardiovascular disease. The approach has face validity. For example, one regularly encounters typical obsessional personalities or avoidant personalities. Personality typologies generate operational criteria. They are useful in research and in operationalising personality disorder diagnoses, and this is the approach used in ICD 10 and DSM IV.

The problem with categorical models of personality is that they fail to describe the full diversity of personality and personality disorders. When diagnostic criteria are applied to populations of patients, some people meet criteria for more than one specific personality disorder, whilst others meet the general criteria for personality disorder, without meeting the criteria for any specific category.

Structural models

These models rest on the hypothetical existence of underlying personality structures that determine behavioural responses. Both psychoanalysis and CBT use implicit structural models.

According to psychoanalysis, personality mainly consists of unconscious structures and mechanisms generated by childhood experience through, for example, the resolution of unconscious conflicts and the formation of internal parental objects. CBT, on the other hand, rests on the belief that behaviour is determined by learned cognitive attitudes to oneself and the world, which lead to rapid automatic thoughts beyond awareness.

Both these traditions have produced concepts of enduring importance in understanding personality development. They share a weakness in that it is difficult to verify that these structures exist. CBT enjoys greater credibility than psychoanalysis, as the efficacy of the associated treatment is more readily demonstrable.

the person will be able to respond adaptively to novel situations and to stresses. People with personality disorder have a limitation in their behavioural repertoire, so that their responses in some (or most) situations are maladaptive.

ICD 10 defines personality disorder thus:

... deeply ingrained and enduring behavioural patterns, manifesting themselves as inflexible responses to a broad range of personal and social situations. They represent either extreme or significant deviations from the way the average individual in a given culture perceives, thinks, feels and particularly relates to others. Such behaviour patterns tend to be stable and to encompass multiple domains of behaviour and psychological functioning. They are frequently, but not always, associated with various degrees of subjective distress and problems in social functioning and performance.

It is apparent that there is not a clear-cut difference between normal and disordered personality. Personality disorder may only become manifest when the environment makes demands the person cannot meet. For example, some impulsive aggressive young men, with a need for external structure and controls, function well in the army, but fall into a chaotic, aimless and delinquent lifestyle on returning to civilian life.

In the light of the competing models, the lack of pathognomnic features, and the use of normative concepts such as 'maladaptive', it is understandable that, from the psychiatric point of view, the whole area of personality is ambiguous and difficult. It is clear that the potential for making errors in assessing personality is considerable. There is a particular risk of deciding that anyone who is unpleasant, or who is disliked by the psychiatrist, has a personality disorder, and that they are therefore beyond psychiatric assistance and can be excluded from treatment. This strategy is particularly seductive because it solves a problem for the psychiatrist.

Box 15.2 sets out a simple framework for thinking about personality development. It is not a model in itself and it is not sophisticated. We have found it useful clinically in linking current problems with historical factors that may have shaped personality. It has the advantage of being consistent with what is known about personality development without demanding a theoretical allegiance to any specific model.

BOX 15.2 Personality development

- A neonate is not a blank sheet. People are born displaying broad temperamental characteristics, which are stable in childhood and beyond. Personality is partly constitutional. However, the existence of these persistent characteristics does not imply that personality is fixed from birth. They are considerably modified by both positive and negative environmental influences.

- These temperamental characteristics profoundly affect parental, especially maternal, behaviour. A mother handles each of her children differently. The child is not a passive recipient of parenting. Child and parent shape each other's behaviour.

- Personality develops through the child's responses to a series of developmental challenges. These arise both biologically (because the child is growing and its capabilities are enlarging) and environmentally (because it encounters new situations which demand responses outside of its current repertoire). Early in life these are simple but profound challenges, such as coping with being wet and hungry. They become progressively more demanding and complex, for example coping with being left at a nursery in the care of strangers. These challenges come thick and fast in early years and more slowly with age. They continue throughout life into old age. For example, many old people face the novel challenge of adjusting to the death of a spouse.

- These challenges proceed in a stepwise fashion and they are repetitive. For example, there are recurrent challenges requiring increasing degrees of independence. These first arise in early childhood as the baby is left with minders and recur when the child goes to school, when the adolescent leaves school, leaves home, gets married and so on.

- It is the resolution of the difficulties caused by each of these challenges that creates new behavioural responses and shapes the available behavioural repertoire of personality. The quality and range of new behaviours depends in part upon the child's constitutional capabilities and in part upon environmental factors, particularly parental behaviour. Not all children are capable of developing all possible behaviours. The resolution of later challenges depends crucially on the quality of the response to earlier challenges. For example, the anxious child of an insecure mother may scream when attempts are made to leave her with strangers, distressing the mother. If the mother responds to her own distress by protecting the child from being left, the child learns to cope with abandonment by alarming her mother. This represents the child's developmental response to this challenge. However, the child has not learned to cope with separations. The child is ill-equipped for future similar experiences such as school. She is likely to be anxious or to refuse school. The problem amplifies over the years.

- If developmental challenges arise prematurely, or if the child has to find a response to abuse (emotional, physical or sexual) and if the child is exposed to other types of adverse experience (such as early loss of a parent), it may develop behaviours which are adaptive in the short term, but which lead to later developmental problems. For example, a child who experiences the loss of a parent may take on a role of caring for her siblings. The child may display a precocious maturity and independence, and adults may praise this. In the long run, she becomes guilty about fulfilling her own needs and grows up to be unable to form close relationships other than in the role of a carer.

- Personality is not solely built from learned behavioural responses. There is an important contribution to personality from ideas that we develop about who we are and the nature of our relationship with the rest of the world. This is, in the broadest sense, the sense of self. It has both profound existential components and more superficial, interpersonal, elements. It determines our self-esteem and self-confidence. An insecure, unloved sense of self can, for example, be found amongst anxious avoidant women and aggressive jealous men.

Assessing personality

Given that most people are not able to give a clear account of their own personality, assessing personality is based on four sources of information:
- The recognition of patterns of behaviour from the history
- Collateral information (from friends or family)
- Records (school reports, social services records, GP records etc.)
- The interaction between patient and psychiatrist

Naturally, it is not necessary or desirable to access all these sources of information for every patient. According to how important or difficult the personality issues are, one moves progressively down this list.

The recognition of patterns of behaviour as the history unfolds is straight-forward, if you know what you are looking for. For example, hints that the person is an anxious perfectionist suggest that they might be markedly obsessional. This then becomes an hypothesis, and one looks for evidence of attachment to routines, dislike of change, intolerance of ambiguity, checking behaviour and so on. If this is not volunteered, it is reasonable to probe:

'Do you like a well-ordered routine?'

'Do you dislike untidiness?'

'Is it difficult to finish things unless they are just right?'

'Do you like to check things? Does this annoy other people?'

These are leading questions, and you have to be careful not to lead the patient into a false positive response. However, the technique will often expose behaviour and personality characteristics which would not have been volunteered, either because their relevance is not obvious (why would anyone think that a lifelong habit of avoiding stepping on the cracks between paving stones was relevant to anorexia nervosa?) or because of embarrassment (how many adults will spontaneously disclose to a stranger that they still avoid stepping on cracks between paving stones?).

The hypothesis must be open to refutation as well as confirmation. If the other features are not present then the hypothesis must fall, but even if all features *are* present there must be evidence that they are lifelong and continuous, or at least that they repeatedly arise under similar circumstances.

It is experience and interviewing hundreds of people that teaches you most about personality and the range of features that tend to cluster together. A lot of women with marked obsessional traits have to make sure that their shoes are kept in neat rows, carefully lined up with each other. This is not in the text books but can be learnt from talking to patients. However, in the first instance, the best source of information is the personality typologies in ICD 10 and DSM IV (American Psychiatric Association, 1994), and other reasonably understandable material about personality problems (for example, Cleckley, 1988).

People who routinely behave badly towards other people tend not to say so. They tend to rationalise their own behaviour and blame everyone else. However, this is not the main reason for wanting to speak to family and friends. People who are exploitative or aggressive or otherwise pathologically self-centred usually expose this by the self-pitying way that they talk about themselves (usually as implausibly unfortunate life-long victims) and about others (who are reported to be uniformly unreliable and uncaring). The point about informants is that they have a clearer understanding of the person's habitual interpersonal behaviour. The psychiatrist will invariably have formed a hypothesis about the patient's personality from the initial interview, and talking to informants allows this to be tested and/or refined. However, in the area of personality, informants are particularly likely to come with an axe to grind, for example to emphasise their opinion that the person is ill and that the behaviour is not their fault or to offer a causational theory ('His mother had a terrible shock when she was pregnant'). It is especially important here to ask what the patient actually does.

It has become increasingly difficult to access old records in recent years. Of course, one needs the patient's permission to do so, but many records seem to have been destroyed. Some institutions, such as certain types of schools, have become very nervous over allegations of child abuse in the distant past, or even of a failure to take action over evidence of child abuse by third parties. This means that precisely the kind of records that you most want to see are the most difficult to obtain. Nonetheless, it is still worth the effort. Contemporaneous accounts are invaluable and tend to provide a wealth of information, even when they are relatively banal records of an unremarkable school career.

The final source of information is the effect that the patient has on the interviewer. This is both a direct reflection of the way that the person interacts and potentially seriously misleading. The trouble is that there are two personalities in the room. If a patient rapidly irritates you, this may say something about their interactions or it may mean you are in a bad mood. As a consequence, the whole approach demands a high level of awareness on the part of the psychiatrist as to the types of patients that they like or dislike, and an appreciation of the impact that their own personality has on the patient. Certainly, before one concludes that some reaction in oneself is a consequence of the patient's personality, it is important to check whether they have the same effect on other people. (As a trainee, a long time ago, one of us was very irritated by a psychotherapist, who recurrently fell asleep during supervision. On being woken, he would explore what it was about the trainee that had made him fall asleep. We were shocked to hear of a recent example of exactly the same behaviour by a much younger psychotherapist.) It is important to bear in mind that one doctor's charming rogue can be another doctor's vicious psychopath.

Having decided that the patient definitely has a personality problem (whether this is a personality disorder or some aspect of their personality that is causing them difficulties), a personality diagnosis can feel rather like a full stop. Identification of the problem, and naming it, provides little useful information about the way forward. It can be more helpful to think about what it is that the patient cannot do. Sometimes, it is possible to work out in this way what has gone wrong developmentally. Using the framework in Box 15.2, one can sometimes further link this with childhood events, as illustrated in Box 15.3.

This process is useful because it does have a degree of predictive power with regard to the types of situation that the person is likely to find difficult in future. However, not everyone who has a difficult childhood develops a personality disorder, and sometimes very disturbed personalities show little evidence of troubled childhoods. The relationship between personality development and adversity is not algebraic.

Some pitfalls in assessing personality

If we assume that the psychiatrist can overcome the temptation to use the diagnosis of personality disorder as a weapon against the patient (a temptation that we would like to think operates at an unconscious level), there are still some further pitfalls in assessment.

The first trap is to base the assessment of personality solely upon the patient's behaviour in a special setting. Experience of a person in a single context, no matter how lengthy, can be misleading. This is especially true during inpatient admissions. Everyone's behaviour in the role of inpatient is altered. For example, during a stay on an orthopaedic ward, you are removed from normal daily responsibilities. You are unable to make choices about daily activities and routine. You are dependent on others for basic needs. You must cope with protracted boredom. As a consequence, a range of regressed behaviour is likely to emerge,

BOX 15.3 A personality problem

Wayne is a 25-year-old man whose wife has thrown him out of the family home. He misses her and their two small children. His wife wants the marriage to continue, but she can no longer tolerate his jealousy and violence.

Wayne's father was a merchant seaman. He was absent from the household for long periods. Wayne, as the eldest of four siblings, was close to his mother, a chronically depressed woman who confided in him. When he was at home, his father drank heavily, and sometimes he beat his wife. Wayne was frightened of his father, and he was distressed at the violence he witnessed. At the same time, like all children, he craved his father's approval.

Wayne learned that discord in relationships was intensely threatening. His parents' relationship provided no model for conflict resolution. Consequently, he was an anxious child, but he followed the model of male behaviour provided by his father. Bravado and aggression eased his fearfulness. He was a bully at school.

Wayne had an intense but insecure dependency on his mother. He rapidly responded with aggression in any situation that he found threatening. As a teenager, he had his mother's name tattooed on his arm, which gave him a sense of her presence.

Wayne has brought an insecure dependency to his relationship with his wife. Although devoted to her and the children, he easily feels that the relationship is under threat. This expresses itself as jealousy, a fear that she is insufficiently attached to him to resist sexual advances from other men. Although he knows that this is destroying the relationship, he cannot prevent himself from doubting her fidelity. In the absence of an alternative strategy to cope, he drinks heavily. As he becomes more intoxicated and disinhibited, his restraint fails and he interrogates his wife. When she becomes exasperated, he takes it as confirmation of his insecurities and the result is aggression and violence.

It is thus possible to link Wayne's current problems to their developmental antecedents. This creates a plausible picture of his personality difficulties, which can be used to both understand the problem and to develop strategies to help him to contain his behaviour. However, a psychiatrist assessing him would not be able to directly obtain this history. For example, if Wayne is asked about his personality, he might describe himself as caring but short-tempered. Asked about his family background, he is likely to describe his mother as a wonderful mum. He may say that he has never been close to his father because he was away at sea for most of his childhood. All of this is true, but it omits the key qualities of the family environment. A psychiatrist interviewing Wayne would be aware that jealousy and aggression are likely to be related to insecure dependency, and would form a hypothesis to this effect. His answers to simple questions would be insufficient to test the hypothesis. The psychiatrist would have to probe about actual family behaviour, for example, about the differences in family life when his father was at sea and when his father was at home. It would be necessary to interview Wayne's wife or his mother in order to establish the continuity of his behaviour patterns from childhood through adulthood.

including childish pranks, vexatious disputes over trivia, bullying and so on. This gives an impression of grossly immature personality. However, the behaviour is determined by the situation and it is not characteristic of fixed behavioural patterns elsewhere. The factors determining regressed behaviour are just as powerful on psychiatric wards, and a judgement made on the basis of inpatient behaviour alone can be expected to be inaccurate.

The second trap arises out of the complex interaction between personality characteristics and substance misuse. On the one hand, some personality disorders are associated with substance misuse. On the other hand, intoxication, especially with alcohol, can release a range of maladaptive behaviours, including aggression, impulsivity and recurrent self-harm in the absence of major personality pathology. People who are intoxicated when interviewed can appear personality disordered, especially if the intoxication is not noticed by the clinician. Intoxication with stimulants, such as amphetamine or cocaine, can make some otherwise reasonable people remarkably unpleasant. Where there is substance abuse, assessment of personality should proceed with caution.

The third trap is due to the effects of affective disorder. Both depression and mania can persist for long periods and profoundly alter behavioural patterns. Hypomania is a term that has no fixed definition, but to us its use should be restricted to describing those states where people are elated and disinhibited without displaying florid overactivity or manic thought disorder. The condition is obvious if you have known the person in the past, as the change in their entire demeanour is dramatic, but to strangers they can simply seem feckless or attention-seeking or arrogant. Mistaking hypomania for personality disorder is one of the commoner errors that we have encountered and made. Depression can also be less than obvious, and a similar mistake can be made. Both errors are less likely if an informant history is available, but this trap never fully goes away, and it is particularly important to recognise and acknowledge that you have made the error once new information becomes available.

Some specific personality disorders

There are some tricky issues associated with particular personality diagnoses. Each new edition of the major diagnostic systems reframes the categories, successive euphemisms are introduced for the most pejorative labels, and diagnostic fashions change, partly in response to alterations in the conceptualisation of different categories. The move away from basing personality diagnoses on speculative theories and towards more objective descriptive groupings is undoubtedly a positive development. However, the overall schema remains puzzling and problematic.

Borderline personality

This diagnostic category has its origins in psychoanalysis, mainly in the USA. Twenty-five years ago, the concept of borderline personality was not generally accepted by psychiatrists in the UK. Today, it is the commonest personality diagnosis applied to women. Conversely, hysterical personality (now known as histrionic personality) was common then and now appears to have virtually disappeared. Box 15.4 sets out the ICD 10 criteria for the two diagnoses. It is obvious that there is a good deal of overlap between them.

It is hardly surprising that these diagnoses are rarely applied to men, as they closely parallel the sexist stereotypes that saloon bar bigots apply to young women

---

BOX 15.4 ICD 10 borderline and histrionic personalities

Emotionally unstable personality disorder, borderline type

'A personality disorder in which there is a marked tendency to act impulsively without consideration of the consequences, together with affective instability. The ability to plan ahead may be minimal, and outbursts of intense anger may often lead to violence or "behavioural explosions"; these are easily precipitated when impulsive acts are criticised or thwarted by others. (*There is a*) general theme of impulsiveness and lack of self control. (*In the* borderline *subtype*) several characteristics of emotional instability are present; in addition the patient's own self-image, aims and internal preferences (including sexual) are often unclear or disturbed. There are usually chronic feelings of emptiness. A liability to become involved in intense and unstable relationships may cause repeated emotional crises and may be associated with excessive efforts to avoid abandonment and a series of suicidal threats or acts of self-harm (although these may occur without obvious precipitants)'.

Histrionic personality disorder

Characterised by

- Self-dramatisation, theatricality, exaggerated expression of emotions;
- Suggestibility, easily influenced by others or circumstances;
- Shallow and labile affectivity;
- Continual seeking for excitement, appreciation by others, and activities in which the patient is the centre of attention;
- Inappropriate seductiveness in appearance or behaviour;
- Over-concern with physical attractiveness;
- Associated features may include egocentricity, self-indulgence, continuous longing for appreciation, feelings that are easily hurt, persistent manipulative behaviour to achieve own needs.

in general. In fact, one does encounter males with these characteristics. However, men in general tend to cope with emotional distress by drinking, violence or both. Consequently, men with these problems tend to be categorised as criminals, alcoholics or psychopaths.

There is a range of overlapping personality disorder typologies (not all of which are in ICD 10), all of which turn on the theme of an inability to sustain close relationships. This includes narcissistic, paranoid, borderline and hysterical personalities. Narcissistic and paranoid can be thought of as nastier (and therefore male) variants of borderline and hysterical. Narcissistic and borderline can be thought of as more poorly integrated personality types than hysterical or paranoid. In psychoanalytic theory, this relates to differences in the robustness of the person's sense of self.

Psychopathic personality

The term 'psychopath' is the most stigmatising diagnostic label available in psychiatry, with a strong implication of dangerousness and untreatability. The term has defied efforts to replace it with a succession of euphemisms, most recently 'dissocial personality disorder' (see Box 15.5). Women are less likely to be given this label than men.

These criteria are wide and embrace a range of types of antisocial people. Almost all unpleasant violent men meet these criteria. There are other ways of understanding antisocial personalities, most of which derive from the work of the late Hervey Cleckley. The modern Hare Psychopathy Checklist (Hare, 1991) is largely based on Cleckley's ideas. Although serious aggression is undoubtedly

---

BOX 15.5 ICD 10 definition of dissocial personality disorder

(A) personality disorder usually coming to attention because of a gross disparity between behaviour and the prevailing social norms, and characterised by:

- Callous unconcern for the feelings of others;
- Gross and persistent attitude of irresponsibility and disregard for social norms, rules and obligations;
- Incapacity to maintain enduring relationships, though having no difficulty in establishing them;
- Very low tolerance to frustration and a low threshold for discharge of aggression, including violence;
- Incapacity to experience guilt and to profit from experience, particularly punishment;
- Marked proneness to blame others, or to offer plausible rationalisations, for the behaviour that has brought the patient into conflict with society.
- There may also be persistent irritability as an associated feature.

BOX 15.6 Cleckley's characteristic features of psychopathy

- Superficial charm and good 'intelligence';
- Absence of delusions and other signs of irrational thinking;
- Absence of nervousness or psychoneurotic manifestations;
- Unreliability;
- Untruthfulness and insincerity;
- Lack of remorse or shame;
- Inadequately motivated antisocial behaviour;
- Poor judgement and failure to learn by experience;
- Pathological egocentricity and incapacity for love;
- General poverty in major affective reactions;
- Specific loss of insight;
- Unresponsiveness in general interpersonal relations;
- Fantastic and uninviting behaviour when drunk and sometimes even when not drunk;
- Suicide rarely carried out;
- Sex life impersonal, trivial and poorly integrated;
- Failure to follow any life plan.

---

a feature of psychopathy, it is not invariable, and there is a range of other features which characterise a narrower, more specific concept of psychopathy. Hervey Cleckley was largely responsible for the popularisation of the concept of multiple personality disorder, and one cannot uncritically embrace his more theoretical ideas. Nonetheless, his book 'The Mask of Sanity' (Cleckley, 1988) is beautifully written and remains the best available descriptive account of the behaviour of psychopaths (Box 15.6).

You do encounter Cleckley-psychopaths, and they are very puzzling and difficult to help. We have found familiarity with his ideas to be helpful. Some psychopaths are obviously and chillingly callous and indifferent. The majority are not. Most psychopaths are capable of convincing expressions of remorse. They not only express guilt for their misdeeds, they also explain why their behaviour was inappropriate. The startling feature is their complete inability to use this knowledge to avoid repetitions of the behaviour and its unwelcome consequences. Their callousness is inferred from what they do rather than being evident from what they say. Over time, one gains the impression that their utterances are entirely an attempt to provoke a reaction in the listener, rather than a reflection of what they genuinely feel. Indeed, it can appear that their feelings are completely disconnected from their thinking. Superficial charm is a common, though not invariable, feature. This sits bizarrely with their evident lack of empathy for anyone else. It is extremely difficult to understand their motivations, and much of their behaviour appears totally irrational. This contrasts with their plausible rationalisations.

Some extremely violent and unpleasant people have clearly developed dissocial personality disorder as a consequence of appallingly abusive childhood experiences. This is not necessarily true of the more narrowly defined psychopath. Even after extensive investigation of their early history, it can be impossible to identify convincing developmental antecedents to explain such a severe disorder of personality functioning. Needless to say, this diagnosis is important, but can only be made with extreme care, as it has far-reaching implications.

Avoidant personality and anankastic (obsessional) personality

These two personality disorders are common. They are both marked by high levels of anxiety and by marked restrictions on the person's day-to-day functioning. However, they are not associated with interpersonal unpleasantness or antisocial behaviour. The important point is that personality disorder is not synonymous with antisocial behaviour. People with these personalities are generally only seen by psychiatrists when they develop another (Axis 1) diagnosis. For this reason, the personality diagnosis is often not made. This does not matter, provided their personality has been understood, as this is important in making a range of judgements.

Schizoid personality

There is considerable confusion over aloof, odd, cerebral people. In recent times, the diagnosis of schizoid personality seems to have fallen out of fashion. The concept of schizotypal personality has been isolated and removed from the schizoid rubric altogether (schizotypal disorder is understood to be essentially forme fruste schizophrenia, with a degree of thought disorder and abnormal affect, but no florid schizophreniform symptoms). However, the decline in the use of the diagnosis of schizoid personality appears to have paralleled the rapid increase of interest in Asperger's syndrome.

Asperger's syndrome can be understood as a mild form of autism, not meeting the full criteria for that disorder, and without a significant impairment of intelligence. The condition definitely exists, and there have always been patients within the general psychiatric population who suffer from it (albeit frequently unrecognised in the past). However, although diagnostic checklists exist, the concept has no clear boundaries. It is assumed to have a constitutional rather than acquired cause, and to be a neuro-developmental disorder. It is going to be important to find a way to distinguish schizoid personality from Asperger's syndrome if we are going to avoid continuing confusion and faddishness in our understanding of how best to help people with these problems. Unfortunately, psychiatry seems to be accumulating an increasing number of diagnostic concepts of uncertain validity, for example, attention deficit disorder in adults.

Main points in this chapter

1. Assessment of personality is a key component of all psychiatric assessments. However, not all clinical situations demand a comprehensive assessment of the patient's personality.
2. In assessing personality, it is useful to have a developmental perspective, whereby current problems can be linked to their historical antecedents. This can help in understanding the patient and in predicting future behaviour.
3. Assessment of personality is rarely possible from a single interview or one source of information. A personality hypothesis has to be developed and tested.
4. There is continuing conceptual confusion about personality and personality disorder, and new ways of thinking about particular clusters of behaviour continue to develop.
5. The diagnosis of personality disorder can be misused to exclude unpopular patients from treatment. Whilst some people cannot be helped, diagnosis should not be used to solve problems for the psychiatrist.
6. Not all people with personality disorder are antisocial, unpleasant or, for that matter, untreatable.

16

Risk and safety

Thirty years ago, psychiatry was the focus of a storm of controversy. Anthony Clare's classic apologia for the profession was entitled 'Psychiatry in Dissent' (Clare, 1980), and this captured the mood of the time. Since the mid-1990s there has been a remarkable rapprochement among the various interest groups that comprise the mental health community. Whilst there are real areas of continuing concern and disagreement, nonetheless, there is a broad consensus over the most helpful types of mental health services, and over the most appropriate type of relationship between service users, carers, statutory services and the voluntary sector. Discourse is no longer dominated by recrimination.

However, there is one area of continuing conflict, and this is the question of risk and how best it should be managed. There is an unresolved tension between policy makers and the media on the one hand, and most of the mental health community on the other (though views within the mental health community vary considerably). As a consequence, issues of risk and safety cause clinicians a good deal of anxiety. Unfortunately, there is little common sense in the debate, and much of the received wisdom is either questionable or plainly wrong. For example, it seems obvious that risk assessment is the key task in avoiding adverse events, when in fact it has a limited role owing to the lack of reliable predictive factors. Multidisciplinary discussion of risk across the largest possible range of agencies sounds like a good idea, but there are cogent arguments that group processes can take over and distort conclusions. The existence of an inexorable rise in the number of violent offences committed by mentally ill people owing to the failure of care in the community is an item of faith in the public debate, but stands in stark contrast to the known facts (Mullen *et al.*, 2000).

In expressing scepticism over risk assessment, we would not wish to be accused of being complacent about risk. One has to acknowledge at the outset that mental health services have a duty to try to prevent bad things happening to their patients and to those around them. Whilst adverse events cannot be wholly eliminated, one has to acknowledge that sometimes this duty is not properly discharged by individual professionals or by whole services. The point of this chapter is not to attack risk assessment and risk management as concepts, but to understand them properly in the interest of optimal safety.

Prediction

Predicting the behaviour of individual human beings is difficult. When psychiatrists try to make detailed predictions of their patients' behaviour, they tend to end up looking foolish. The only half-way reliable predictor of future behaviour is past behaviour. The whole field of forensic psychiatry is based on this psychological principle, which can be summarised as '*he might do it again*'. Unfortunately, this offers little assistance when attempting to assess whether people are likely to behave in undesirable ways for the first time, which is the type of risk that community psychiatrists most frequently have to worry about.

It is true that there are a number of risk factors that are known to increase the likelihood of certain types of adverse events. For example, young males who have an alcohol problem are very much more likely to behave violently than the rest of the population. This is as true of the mentally ill as it is of the general population. The broad risk factors for violence, suicide and homicide are not changed by the presence or absence of mental illness. However, the large majority of people with the relevant risk factors never display adverse behaviours, and some people who do act in undesirable ways, do so in the absence of any relevant risk factor. Risk factors have a limited utility in predicting individual behaviour. This is bound to be true when a much larger number of people are affected by the risk factors than will ever carry out an adverse behaviour.

In the UK, the whole question of mental illness and risk became a matter of widespread public concern following a series of events culminating in the Clunis report (Ritchie *et al.*) in 1994. This report explored the treatment of a mentally ill man who was well-known to mental health services in London, and who eventually killed a stranger, Jonathan Zito, at a tube station. There have been numerous subsequent reports on similar tragedies. These reports are in the public arena, and perusal of them is depressing, as they reveal repetitive themes. Few of these homicides could have been predicted. However, many of them might have been prevented if services had avoided certain key failings, namely:
- failure to collate information properly;
- failure to communicate adequately;
- failure to interview informants;
- failure to assertively follow-up evasive and aggressive patients;
- making assumptions about patients (for example, in the case of Christopher Clunis, a young black man, it was assumed that he was a drug user and that he was out of touch with his family, neither of which was true);

- re-diagnosing aggressive patients (in a number of cases, aggressive patients who actually suffered from a treatable mental illness, such as schizophrenia, were re-diagnosed as suffering from untreatable personality disorder or self-inflicted drug-induced psychosis and excluded from services).

What this tends to suggest is that, whilst it may be difficult to predict adverse events, it may be possible to avoid them by observing the basic principles of good psychiatric practice. This includes being prepared to deal with unlikeable and difficult patients, as they are often at the greatest risk.

The nature of risk in psychiatry

Risk in psychiatry has a number of particular features:
- Risk in psychiatry is not a continuous quantifiable variable.
- It is much easier to say that a risk is 'high' than that it is 'low'.
- The risks faced by people with mental illness are heterogeneous.
- Reducing one type of risk sometimes increases other types of risks.
- There are risks to patients, to those around them and to the clinician (if he fails to prevent adverse events).
- Adverse events occur with a low frequency in each clinician's working life.
- Clinicians are exposed to small numbers of 'high risk' patients and large numbers of 'low risk' patients. They will therefore encounter more adverse events amongst 'low risk' patients.

Actuarial versus contextual risk

Risk in psychiatry is profoundly affected by a multitude of contextual factors. In the absence of reliable predictors, people cannot be put into high, medium and low risk categories that can be defined by actuarial probabilities. Risk is dynamic, and rests upon an interplay between the individual's personality, the features of their illness and the situation that they find themselves in. Although there is a small group of people who can justifiably be described as dangerous (because they are likely to remain liable to do dangerous things in the long term), more commonly dangerousness is not embedded in the person, but in the total situation. For example, an aggressive young man with an alcohol problem may only become dangerous when he develops jealous delusions about a girlfriend who, by virtue of her own alcohol problem, does not take action to protect herself from his aggression.

It is very difficult to say that risk is low. The absence of positive risk factors does not indicate safety, and there are even fewer reliable protective factors than risk factors. It is psychologically more difficult to say that someone is safe.

If you say that someone is at high risk and nothing happens, then you have been effective in containing risk. If you say someone is, at low risk and something happens, then you are just wrong. Risk can change quite quickly, and a 'low risk' label can be just as problematic as a 'high risk' label. However, unless the majority of people are regarded as 'low risk', the term 'high risk' is completely meaningless.

Heterogeneity of risk

We tend to think of risk mainly in terms of suicide, violence, self-neglect and vulnerability to exploitation. However, there is a wide range of things that can go wrong in the life of a person with mental illness. For example, noticeably bizarre behaviour may carry little direct risk to the patient or those around him, but may carry a high risk of harm due to the reactions of others. If you look peculiar and persistently hang about near a school, there is a real risk of becoming a victim of serious violence, owing to public anxieties about predatory paedophiles.

Psychiatrists have traditionally tended to focus on those risks that arise directly out of the patient's mental illness, for example, the risks arising from suicidal thoughts as a consequence of depression, or homicidal ideas as a consequence of delusions. However, not all risks to mentally ill people are a direct consequence of the illness itself. For example, unpleasant and violent men can develop schizophrenia, and they may remain violent and unpleasant irrespective of their mental state. The extent to which mental health services should take responsibility for containing such risks is highly contentious. A pedantic separation of behaviours into those related and those unrelated to mental illness is not always realistic. Many risk behaviours are mediated by the common non-specific factor of impaired judgement. It is not always appropriate to relieve mentally ill people of responsibility for their actions. However, the relationship between mental state and risk can be difficult to pick apart.

The balance of risks

Action to avoid one type of risk can increase other types of risks. Clearly, a failure to detect or take notice of suicidal thoughts can mean that the patient comes to harm or dies. However, overreacting to fleeting and resisted suicidal ideas can lead to an excessively restrictive, custodial style of care, which itself can inflict real social harm, and may impede recovery. Most of the time, dealing with risk is about balancing competing concerns over different types of risks. The clinician has to be prepared to take decisive action when the apparent risk is too great to tolerate, and has to retain a sense of proportion over the seriousness and likelihood of different types of risks. For example, failure to take action over concerns that a patient will act violently for fear that the therapeutic relationship may be damaged does not represent a proportionate or appropriate weighting of differential risk.

Risk to whom?

Most of the time, psychiatrists are concerned with risk to the patient. However, people who are mentally ill can sometimes represent a danger to those around them in a variety of ways. There are some ways of thinking about risk that shifts the risk around rather than actually reducing risk. Take for example an angry, manic woman recently admitted informally to an acute mental health unit. Patients like this can easily get into conflict with other patients, and there is then a real risk of violence. Going for a walk with a member of staff can defuse the situation and reduce the risk of immediate assault. Such patients can also get into conflict with staff. Sending them for a walk on their own can reduce the sense of tension on the ward, and may help the patient to calm down; equally, it may expose the general public to the risk of assault. In the latter instance, although the measure reduces visible risk, it actually moves the risk from one group of people to another. Furthermore, any risk to other people is also a risk to the patient, who has to live with the consequences. Inpatient staff are trained to deal with aggression, but the general public are not. As a result, assaults in public places often have worse consequences. Overall, the strategy may increase, not diminish, risk.

However, there is a more complex type of third-party risk, which is the risk to the clinician of censure. The objective evidence suggests that risk containment by mental health services has become no worse over recent decades, and it has probably improved. For example, homicides by mentally ill people have decreased since the Second World War, both as a proportion of all homicides and in absolute numbers (Taylor and Gunn, 1999). However, concern over safety has followed a general social trend in developed countries towards increasing intolerance of risk. There is now a backlash against this general trend to the effect that, if a risk-free life were possible (which it is not), such an existence would be bland, boring and ultimately meaningless. Whilst the issue of risk in psychiatry is affected by this wider social debate, we work in an environment where adverse events are closely scrutinised. This has led to a rising fear amongst psychiatrists that they are likely to be held responsible if their patients behave in certain ways, especially if they commit suicide or homicide.

There is, in fact, little or no evidence that psychiatrists are likely to be unfairly criticised by employers or licensing authorities under these circumstances, provided they are conscientious in what they do. The key issue is usually whether decisions were made with reasonable care at the time, rather than whether they were right with the advantage of hindsight. Unfortunately, the press tends not to have a sense of complexity or fair play, and it is probably the real risk of a mauling in the regional or national newspapers that has generated a general twitchiness over risk. As a consequence, risk assessment is sometimes more concerned with protecting the professional than with making judgements in the best interests of the patient and those around him. This has a range of adverse effects, as making risk judgements and tolerating risk is a necessary part of all mental health practice.

Some patients exploit clinicians' anxieties by threatening to harm themselves or other people. This is almost invariably done with the intention of persuading the psychiatrist to do something that he thinks is inappropriate, such as admitting the person to hospital or prescribing abusable drugs. On the one hand, the psychiatrist cannot give in to threats, and compliance to the person's wishes out of fear can only lead to further threats, and to unacceptable practices. On the other hand, this has to be tempered by an awareness that some people, either because of their subculture or because of illness, have a very low threshold for using threats, and that the conflict can reflect the fact that the doctor has made a misjudgement. There is an essential difference between allowing oneself to be manipulated and being prepared to reconsider a decision, despite unreasonable behaviour.

Low-frequency events

One of the problems in trying to prevent low-frequency events is that it is almost impossible to gauge how effective you are. If none of your patients are involved in adverse incidents, you do not know what would have happened if you had not intervened. If your patients *are* involved in such incidents, you do not know how many more would have been if you had done nothing.

Low-frequency events do not happen at regular intervals. They tend to cluster (think of a Geiger counter measuring background radiation; it tends to click sporadically with periods of silence). Most psychiatrists experience occasional 'epidemics' of adverse events amongst their patients. It can be hard to tell whether something has gone systematically wrong with your clinical practice, or whether this is just an artefact of low probability statistics (given that both are possible).

There are relatively few patients in any psychiatrist's case load who are regarded as 'high risk', and conscientious teams put a good deal of effort into these patients. However, there are many 'low risk' patients. If we assume that the assessment of low risk is generally accurate, each individual patient is unlikely to do anything untoward. However, the clinician has a different risk exposure, as contact with a very large number of low-risk patients means that some will be involved in adverse incidents. In fact, given that the average clinician is unlikely to have a patient commit homicide in an entire career, such events are as likely to occur amongst 'low risk' patients as amongst 'high risk' patients.

There are two ways of misinterpreting this. The first misinterpretation is to say that risk assessment is therefore a waste of time. However, there is nothing about these differential probabilities that says it is impossible to avoid adverse events amongst those at high risk. It does explain why adverse events are impossible to completely eliminate.

The second misinterpretation is to conclude that there are no 'low risk' patients and to develop a very cautious style of clinical practice. For example, patients under the care of psychiatrists, as a group, are more likely to kill themselves than other people. You could therefore say that all of your patients are at raised risk, and this would be true. However, attempts to treat all patients as at high risk of suicide would rapidly overwhelm the service, and the lack of a focus on those truly at high risk would make risk management less effective. Such a strategy would be likely to increase, not decrease, the suicide rate amongst psychiatric patients. An overzealous, custodial and restrictive pattern of care would also be likely to deter people from seeing psychiatrists, which in all probability would eventually increase the rate of suicide amongst the general population.

There is a final twist to the question of 'low risk': taking a small risk repeatedly with an individual patient can be dangerous, as the risk event is then much more likely to happen to that patient. It is important to recognise the difference between the psychiatrist and the patient being repeatedly exposed to a relatively small risk.

Risk assessment

'Risk assessment' is a concept of ambiguous meaning in psychiatry, but there is no alternative but to use it, as it is the standard term. It involves a process of critically weighing objective and subjective factors at a particular point in time.

The cornerstone of risk assessment, and of all clinical practice, is having access to accurate and comprehensive information. Without a proper history, it is impossible to assess risk. However, access to information can be difficult, particularly since modern case notes are extremely bulky and invariably run to multiple volumes. The most important part of risk assessment is collating all the information.

It is possible to trawl case notes, or the history that the patient gives, for risk factors. These include evidence of previous aggression or suicidality, evidence of impulsivity and lack of restraint, evidence of substance misuse, evidence of social isolation and a lack of social relationships, low self-esteem and an unusually strong interest in depictions of violence. This type of risk factor is relatively non-specific, but increases the risk for adverse behaviours in general. There are much more specific risk factors, which are discussed below, and which carry a relatively heavy weighting for concern.

However, there is another process in assessing risk, equally dependent on good quality information, but requiring a more analytical approach. Patients' life histories can be understood as a narrative, and mental illness is part of that narrative. Events do not just happen to people. We all have long-term patterns and cycles of behaviour, and life histories unfold and develop. Both episodes in people's lives and whole life histories have a trajectory, a general direction of movement. This may coincide with the person's explicit intentions, but may be completely independent of any plans or deliberate actions they take. Spotting the trajectory of a developing situation can be critical in preventing adverse events. For example, some patients show signs of heading towards a suicide attempt without ever acknowledging such an intention. A middle-aged divorced man who is depressed after losing his job, who then gives up his social activities and gives away a much loved pet is clearly moving towards a suicide attempt, whether he has a formed intention or not. Spotting such trajectories is one of the reasons why histories need to be pieced together in such a way as to make sense from a psychological point of view.

People who are planning to do something will often say so. There is every reason to ask people about their intentions. Of course, some patients claim to be suicidal in order to manipulate the questioner, but it is usually possible to distinguish the two situations on the basis of contextual factors. Although all doctors are taught to ask depressed people about suicidal ideas, there is a greater reluctance to discuss aggressive feelings. Conversely, many psychiatrists in training seem to learn to indiscriminately ask patients 'Do you ever feel like killing anyone?', which naturally invites the response 'Yes, you'. It is not difficult to ask about aggression in a stepwise fashion; questions about irritability provide a useful probe. When asking about both suicidal and aggressive feelings, it can be important not to accept blunt denials immediately. A little more probing ('are you sure?') often reveals feelings that people are reluctant to disclose.

There is a surprising general reluctance amongst psychiatrists to share concerns over risk with patients. In general, one can learn more about the risk if one explains one's concerns to the patient. The risk does, after all, belong primarily to the patient, who therefore has a right to know about it. Furthermore, patients are routinely very helpful partners in devising risk containment strategies, including when the risk is of violence.

Risk assessment instruments

These days, most services have a risk assessment instrument that some member of the team is expected to complete. These instruments are something of a mixed blessing. Most services devise their own risk assessment instrument, because there are no validated and reliable instruments suitable for general use. If risk assessment rests mainly on the completion of such an instrument, generating a risk rating, then it is likely to be a poor-quality exercise. Risk assessment is never a completed task, but needs to be thought about constantly. These instruments can only generate a very general indication of risk, and they cannot deal with the full range of potential risks (which is extremely wide). They are only as reliable as the information that is put into them. They do not encourage the exploration of trajectory. However, they do create an awareness of risk, and, as they are effectively checklists for risk factors, they do encourage thorough information gathering. We are doubtful of their true value, but they are currently in vogue and they will probably be with us for some time. Provided they are neither regarded as the whole of risk assessment nor given credibility beyond their limited predictive power, they are a useful aid to thoroughness. They are, however, always tedious to complete.

Some pitfalls in risk assessment

The biggest pitfall in risk assessment is the gut feeling, the uneasy sense that the situation is not safe and the converse sense that the situation is safer than it might appear. Gut feelings do sometimes reflect real intuitions over clinical situations. If they are reliable, it should be possible to operationalise and understand them. For example, if someone makes you feel very uneasy, it may be because their eye contact and body language indicate that they are preparing to attack you. In this case, it should be possible to work out what it is about them that makes you uneasy. On the other hand, it may be because they are tall, black and male, and you have a prejudice that large black men are intrinsically dangerous. If gut feelings cannot be operationalised and broken down to constituent parts, then they are very likely to be prejudices.

This would equally apply to a prejudice that well brought up middle class women do not attack doctors (they sometimes do). The patients in whom we are most likely to underestimate risk are those who are most like ourselves and those who we most like. It is important to be objective about risk, and this is best achieved by discussing cases with colleagues, or other team members. This is one of the reasons why all patients should routinely be the subject of team discussion or individual supervision.

However, it is important that, on a case-by-case basis, one clinician holds responsibility for assessing risk, and much of the time this will be the consultant psychiatrist. This is because team decision-making about risk is very vulnerable to uncontrolled group dynamics. Teams can persuade themselves that people are either at much higher or much lower risk than is objectively the case. There are two processes that particularly encourage this. In most teams, team members tend to agree. Therefore, there is a psychological pressure to agree with other team members' assessments. The fact that the rest of the group agrees then reinforces the index team member's conviction of the correctness of their assessment. This tends to lead to reassuring conclusions, as the view that nothing is likely to happen is usually correct, except when it is not. However, the situation can also develop whereby team members can convince themselves that a patient who they do not like is much more dangerous than they really are, and that some other team should be dealing with them.

Risk factors

As stated above, there are a number of non-specific risk factors that are associated with adverse events of all types, and these are largely related to social isolation, dislocation, impulsivity and having nothing to lose. This amounts to anomie, and it is sobering to realise that Durkheim's observations (Durkheim, 1951) remain relevant over a hundred years after their original publication. There are, however, a few more specific risk factors that arise amongst general psychiatric patients (there are others of relevance to, for example, forensic psychiatry, but they are beyond the scope of this book).

Suicide

Suicide does not occur exclusively amongst the mentally ill, but the risk of it is increased by all mental illnesses. If you are diagnosed as suffering from schizophrenia, bipolar affective disorder or anorexia nervosa, then the risk that you will eventually die by your own hand rises to between 8 and 15%. This is clearly a substantial risk, but it is spread over many years, so that the risk that an individual will commit suicide in a given year is relatively low. A strong religious faith or a supportive spouse (especially a wife) reduce the risk, but do not eliminate it. Hopelessness is the critical clinical factor. Patients often do not express hopelessness, but one can infer it. Evidence of sorting out one's affairs, and of preparing the environment for one's death are ominous. People who are depressed and paranoid are particularly likely to take their own life. Physical illness leading to permanent pain and disability are as important as mental illness in increasing individual suicide risk. Some people commit suicide out of anger rather than depression. It can be an act of aggression, designed to hurt specific individuals. It should not be assumed that anger is only associated with violence to others.

In assessing the risk associated with a particular act of self-harm, the degree of lethality of the act is important, but so is the patient's perception of potential lethality. If the patient believed that an overdose of propranolol was likely to be fatal because they are heart tablets, the fact that the overdose was not life-threatening is irrelevant. The patient's attitude to their survival is important. Some acts of self-harm do nothing to alter the patient's situation; some improve their situation; and some make things worse. This is relevant when the person appraises their situation in the light of their survival. If nothing has changed, this affects the risk of recurrence.

It is important to bear in mind that suicide risk is not necessarily at its highest when the illness is most severe. It has long been recognised that people suffering from severe depression often take their lives during the recovery phase, and that people suffering from schizophrenia are at high risk in the first few weeks after discharge from hospital. This demonstrates that suicidality is not just related to mental state abnormalities, but also to wider contextual factors.

Serious aggression

The diagnosis of schizophrenia increases the risk that the person will show serious aggression (Brennan *et al.*, 2000). However, this is an epidemiological finding. The increase in risk is so small that it is irrelevant in assessing individual risk. However, if one leaves aside the general risk factors for aggression (male gender, substance misuse, social dislocation etc.), there are a handful of specific mental state abnormalities that are of relevance to serious aggression. It is well recognised that jealous delusions are particularly likely to lead to violence. The common scenario is that the patient has been interrogating their spouse for months about a supposed infidelity. Eventually, exasperated, the spouse says something like 'OK, have it your own way, I have been having an affair', and the patient then becomes enraged and violent. The traditional advice to spouses who are the subject of jealous delusions is to move out, but this is rarely practical. All such spouses should be warned of the dangers of false confession, even if the apparent danger is small or non-existent.

Jealous delusions are a sub-type of delusions about people in the immediate environment. Such delusions are always of concern. It only makes sense that, if you think you are being persecuted or interfered with by people around you, you will eventually try and sort them out. The closer the relationship with the deluded person, the greater the danger, and the fact that the two people are normally on friendly terms is not reassuring. For example, some people deal with Capgras delusions (that someone close to them has been replaced by a double) by trying to kill the 'replacement' in the hope that the 'original' will return.

Command hallucinations are not necessarily acted upon, and they can be hard to distinguish from obsessional thoughts. However, whenever someone receives hallucinatory instructions, it is important to explore the extent to which the person feels compelled to act on them and whether there are internal restraints against obeying.

Depressed people sometimes develop delusions that it is not just them who are doomed, but those they care about too. They sometimes believe that they have brought shame or disaster on their family, or contaminated them. This can lead to 'mercy killings', usually combined with suicide. It is not only children who are victims of such homicides, but also other vulnerable, dependent people such as elderly parents or disabled spouses.

Driving

The most dangerous weapon that most of us possess is a motor car. Driving when unfit is a major and common risk to patients and the general public. Taking psychotropic medication substantially increases the chances of being involved in a serious accident. All mental illnesses make driving more difficult through impaired concentration, distractions such as hallucinations, impaired judgement and increased impulsivity. Depressed patients sometimes become indifferent to their own safety and drive more recklessly as a form of fatalistic Russian roulette. This is not to say that people with mental illness necessarily should not drive, but their fitness to do so should be assessed, and if they are not fit, they need to be clearly informed of this. It is also important to remember that some people drive without a licence and without owning a car; young men in particular need to be questioned closely as to whether they drive.

Safety considerations

All mental health professionals are shouted at or threatened from time to time. This is an unfortunate but unavoidable aspect of the job. However, actual assaults are relatively rare. In the community, the greatest risk is of having a road traffic accident or of being mugged. Nonetheless, to paraphrase a point made earlier, a low risk taken repeatedly becomes a high risk. There is therefore good reason to be cautious or indeed cowardly. This not only protects you, it also protects the patient. Frightened doctors tend to make bad decisions and patients often pay a heavy price for assaulting mental health staff (insofar as they get sent to secure facilities and are treated as dangerous for ever after).

Although a number of points about safety have been made elsewhere, the main principles in maintaining one's personal safety in hospital and in the community are worth reiterating here. These points cannot always be followed. If you have to break these principles, this should be done as an exercise in calculated risk-taking rather than in a spirit of blind optimism.

- When you first assess a patient, the amount of information available may be quite limited. You should insist that referrers give as much information as possible. Amongst other things, this allows you to be as clear as you can be about risk prior to the interview. If there is cause for concern, gather information about the individual from other professionals and from GP records beforehand. If another agency is involved, and can be contacted without a breach of confidentiality, this should be done before assessment. It is especially important to gather information prior to the first visit to a patient's home. It is sometimes necessary to speak to friends and relatives prior to a home visit, though this can easily compromise confidentiality. Never go into someone's home for clinical purposes without speaking to someone who knows them first. The best protection against unexpected aggression is good quality information.

- Some types of patients are objectively more likely to assault the doctor. People who are aggressive when well are likely to be aggressive when ill, as are patients who are intoxicated with drugs or alcohol. Patients whose psychosis leads them to believe that there is a threat to them in the immediate environment may deal with this through aggression. Patients with delusional ideas that specific individuals are responsible for their misfortunes are likely to react aggressively.

- Before commencing an interview, one should be reasonably certain that the patient is not carrying a weapon. Interviews with aggressive patients should not go ahead if there are objects in the room that can easily be used as weapons, for example, heavy ashtrays or kitchen knives.

- Ensure that you can escape unimpeded. You cannot allow the patient to have control of the space. You should position yourself between the patient and the door. In the patient's own home, ensure that you cannot be locked in.

- Make sure that assistance is available. This means that there must be an agreement between yourself and other staff on how you will raise the alarm, and that they will respond to the alarm. This is reasonably straightforward in a hospital, provided you do not assume that the arrangements are clear without discussing them. The agreement on assistance should be explicitly stated between the staff on hand and yourself.

- When working in the community, either alone or with another team member, make sure that someone knows exactly where you are, and when you are due back. They need to know exactly what to do if you do not arrive. The latter is particularly important, as simply knowing that you are late creates a dilemma for the other person, if there is no agreement as to the threshold for regarding this as an emergency. On the other hand, if you know that the police will be called if you are more than half an hour late, you are unlikely to allow yourself to be delayed.

- Be prepared to withdraw if your fear is rising or if you cannot calm the patient. If the interview is failing, for example if the patient is becoming more threatening, a break will not make things worse, and it sometimes helps.

- In the community, try to work in pairs. In a first assessment in the community, the patient is often reassured by the presence of someone they know. In the hospital, if you do not feel safe alone with the patient, have someone else with you. Make it clear at the outset who is conducting the interview and that the other person should not intervene unless invited to do so. If you are alone and you have to say something that is likely to be provocative, break and get someone else to be with you.

- If you are seeing the patient at home, let them know that you are going to visit. It is unannounced visits that most commonly trigger aggression. If one looks at the situation from the patient's point of view, the unannounced arrival of a psychiatrist at the front door is obviously provocative. If there is a good reason to visit without warning, usually because admission to hospital under compulsion is anticipated, there is no option but to speak to a family member first, even if this compromises confidentiality.

- Travel with the means to summon help, which these days means a mobile phone. This only works if you take care to ensure that the batteries are charged. The sight of a 'dead' mobile phone is little deterrent to the determined assailant.

- Be aware of aspects of your own behaviour that are likely to convey threat to the patient. This means attempting to retain an awareness of the patient's point of view. An angry patient is unlikely to respond well to being told he is going to be detained. Trying to argue with him is likely to be provocative. Tense body language and the invasion of personal space are threatening. Try to adopt a relaxed posture and talk slowly. If you think the patient is being aggressive because of fear, say so. Similarly, aggressive patients are frequently unaware that they are frightening others, and it can be helpful to point this out. An appearance of not listening to what the patient is saying is very frustrating. You may not be able to completely relieve the patient's frustration, but it will ease if they feel that their concerns are being acknowledged.

- Do not take any responsibility for physically restraining the patient unless you have been trained to do this. Hospital nursing staff are trained to do this safely. A preparedness to grab the patient is easily read in body posture, and it does nothing to reassure the patient.
- Most psychiatric services now provide staff with training in 'breakaway techniques'. Attend these courses.
- Do not carry a weapon. Even a can of pepper spray can be turned against you. Producing a weapon is more likely to provoke violence than prevent it.
- A very small number of patients bear a grudge and stalk mental health professionals. It is wise to have an ex-directory telephone number, to use a pseudonym for the electoral register (this is legal in the UK), and to be circumspect in revealing where you live.

Main points in this chapter

1. Predicting behaviour is difficult.
2. Risk assessment depends on collating full and accurate information, on assessing the trajectory of the situations as it develops and on being aware of the major risk factors.
3. Adverse events occur amongst 'low risk' as well as 'high risk' patients.
4. Adverse events are minimised by doing the job properly and by recognising that the patients we least like dealing with are at highest risk.
5. Personal cowardice is the safest policy in the course of a whole career in mental health, despite the fact that the personal risks are small.

17

Note-keeping, letters and reports

At this stage, we hope that the reader is persuaded that psychiatric assessment involves far more than history taking, mental state examination and diagnosis. It is a dynamic process that lays the foundation of a therapeutic alliance. This includes the formation of a shared understanding with the patient of the nature of the problem, set in the meaningful context of the patient's life. This shared understanding does not necessarily arise immediately, and the process of achieving it can take years. On the clinician's part, there has to be a selective and critical approach to the mass of information available. The psychiatrist has to be able to identify the most important features of the overall situation, to recognise patterns of behaviour within the history and to identify the trajectory of the patient's life history. The impact of all this effort is largely lost unless both the facts and the analysis are properly recorded and communicated.

Note-keeping

Once you enter your fifth decade of life, it is very noticeable that nothing is quite as good as it used to be. There can be little doubt that this is predominantly an effect of the ageing process, but in two particular areas, it is quite certain that the perception is correct. You eventually reach a point where you, yourself, are nothing like as good as you used to be; and neither are psychiatric records.

One day, someone in authority will realise that the quality of case notes cannot be measured by their weight. Modern case notes are packed with forms: care programme approach forms, risk assessment forms, photocopies of welfare benefit forms and so on. Whatever the advantages of the use of proformas in general, their bulk is beyond dispute. This means that most people's notes run to multiple volumes, and it is very difficult to retrieve information (indeed, one could argue that risk assessment instruments have become popular in order to record information that was much easier to access before such forms came into use). The plethora of documents can also give a false impression that everything has been recorded and that it is less important than it used to be to keep clear running clinical records, when the opposite is, in fact, the case.

Running notes, made as the interview proceeds, are invaluable. They may be unreadable to everyone other than the author, but this is not a reason not to make them. The main tenets of good record-keeping are simple. Every sheet should be dated and marked with the patient's name, in case they become detached. There should be a record of where the interview happened, and who was present, each person identified both by full name and relationship to the patient/professional role. It is surprising how quickly staff turn over and how quickly everyone forgets, for example, who 'Brian' was. There should be a clear and detailed record of what led up to the patient being seen, especially in emergency situations. The source of information and its perceived reliability should be noted. There should be examples of behaviour and symptoms of concern, as discussed in Chapter 3. There should be a clear distinction made between what has been observed directly, and what has been reported. Sensitive information should be very clearly labelled as such. If an undertaking is made not to disclose information to third parties, this should be conspicuously flagged, and it is usually best to record this on a separate sheet marked 'Not to be disclosed without permission'.

At the end of the note, we are in the habit of having a section for conclusions headed 'Impression'. If some part of this is not disclosed to the patient, it is important to record this, and if third parties are told of conclusions, this too should be noted. We follow this with a heading 'Plan'. It is good practice to have such a section in the notes for every follow-up appointment as well as assessment interviews, so that you have to think about what you are trying to do and so that you notice if the plan goes wrong. The 'plan' section should include an explanation as to why you have made particular decisions. It is inevitable that some short cuts occur in making notes, but some should definitely be avoided. For example, if you are arranging blood tests, there is no point in noting 'routine bloods requested'. Each investigation should be listed, together with the result when it arrives. Similarly, you should record each of the major statements you make and any suggestions you make to the patient. It does not instil great faith if you have to ask the patient what you said or did at the last interview. Finally, each entry should be clearly marked with your name, job title and the team you work with (Box 17.1).

Letters

Letters are a difficult skill to master. They have a dual purpose. They communicate what you intend to do and why to a third party, usually the referrer. They also serve as a legible and clear summary of your findings, your intentions and subsequent events, which forms the chronological spine of the case record.

BOX 17.1 Paper records will always be with us

Over the last twenty-five years, managers of mental health services have resisted improvements to case note systems on the grounds that paper notes will shortly be replaced by electronic record systems. Computers have become ubiquitous, and hard copies of e-mails, faxes and printouts of electronic contact records have added to the bulk of paper notes. Computers suffer from viruses and hackers. Software crashes routinely and the IT department phones to let you know that 'the system is down'. Organisational structures change regularly and, when organisations merge, invariably 'the systems don't talk to each other'. We once laughed at ageing colleagues who were sceptical of new technology. At this late stage, our confidence in the imminent arrival of the comprehensive electronic record system has been somewhat undermined. In fact, we are now quite confident that we will both retire without ever having seen such a system in action. The single most secure piece of advice we can offer in this book is that you should assume that paper records will never disappear.

As such, they need to be processed and thought through documents rather than a simple reiteration of the 'raw' history and mental state examination.

Many services have a computerised template for routine letters and discharge summaries. The intention is to ensure that certain essential information is communicated reliably, and they do achieve this end. However, they militate against the creation of a clear narrative, which is the hallmark of a good clinical letter. Indeed, when reading these templated letters, it is often hard to understand why decisions have been made. For example, when patients are seen by trainees in A&E, there is often a brief letter following a template, which sets out the circumstances of an act of deliberate self-harm and requests a consultant appointment. Without more information, it can be very hard to tell why it was felt that the patient needed to be seen, or to assess which team member might most appropriately see them. Templated letters are certainly better than a poor letter or no letter, but we prefer something less basic.

Clinical letters should tell you why the patient has presented in this way at this time. They should tell the story and be easy to follow. They should not be too long, around two sides of A4 paper for an assessment letter, perhaps one side for a follow-up letter. It should be easy to comprehend why the conclusions were drawn and what the treatment plan is. If the interview has not led to a full history being gathered, it should be clear what is known, but also what still needs to be found out. The test of an adequate letter is that, if you drop dead before the next interview, it should be reasonably straightforward for the next clinician to pick up the threads of the case on the basis of your letter.

Very few GPs will read an assessment letter from start to finish. If you want them to do something (such as organise investigations or prescribe a drug), it needs to be clearly stated at the end of the letter, if necessary in bold type. If there are essential tasks to be carried out, such as monitoring of blood lithium levels, it should be clear as to whether you intend to do this or whether you expect the recipient to carry them out.

Anyone who can write a good assessment letter should be capable of doing well in the related, but slightly different, task of passing clinical post-graduate examinations. Assessments and letter writing is one of the most important ways of preparing for these exams (Box 17.2).

BOX 17.2 A clinical assessment letter about a difficult and fragmentary interview

Dear Dr Patel,

Re: Irene Wright (d.o.b: 18/6/55)

This patient of yours was referred to the CMHT by a student social worker from Child and Family Social Services, Maria Dutton, who has been working with Mrs Wright and her two children since July 2004. I interviewed her with Carol Penley, CPN and Ms Dutton, in clinic on 23/12/04.

The referral did not occur because of a clinical crisis, but because the family have no money to live on, owing to an enormous mix up over their benefits. However, this fortuitously provided an opportunity to carry out a mental health assessment on Mrs Wright. She has been referred to this service on at least three occasions since 1999, but has always declined assessment.

The interview was not 100% satisfactory. There were five of us in the room (Mrs Wright brought her 14-year-old daughter, Emily, with her). We did not obtain a comprehensive history, but did manage to establish the likely nature of the problem.

As I'm sure you are aware, Mrs Wright has a long history of odd behaviour and neglect of her house, with episodes of shouting and verbal abuse. She has always been reluctant to engage with services. In 1996, the Alcohol Dependency Service treated her for three weeks as an inpatient. It is hard to pin down the severity of her alcohol problem in the past. She admits to a lifetime maximum intake of three quarters of a bottle of wine a day, but Maria Dutton is quite certain that her consumption has been closer to a bottle a day quite recently. However, we could find little evidence of physical or social sequelae of heavy drinking. She denies ever having suffered withdrawal symptoms and she has never drunk daily, but she does regard alcohol as a problem to her that she has to keep under control. There was no evidence of alcohol intoxication or withdrawal at interview.

At interview, Mrs Wright was a little dishevelled, with adequate, but not good, self care. Her skin was reddened. She told me that she had been washing her hands with bleach, but the appearance was more suggestive of prolonged exposure to the cold. Her mood was euthymic, and she engaged pleasantly with our group. She did, however, display marked thought disorder of the schizophreniform type, at times to the point of incoherence. There were copious active psychotic symptoms. It is hard to know whether her difficulty in describing these arises from her awareness that they sound very strange. She was certainly quite guarded on some subjects, and sometimes altered her descriptions of symptoms when I tried to clarify their nature. Despite these difficulties, we did establish that she believes that an organisation implanted a probe in her brain when she was an inpatient in 1996, and that she has subsequently been used to transmit messages about forthcoming global disasters. She believes her movements are being monitored. She suffers from continuous auditory hallucinations, and paused to listen to these at several points during the interview. She told us she has to lip-read in order to distinguish speakers' voices from hallucinatory voices. She gave me the impression that she also suffers from somatic hallucinations, passivity experiences and delusions of reference, but it was hard to be certain about this on the basis of this interview. Despite this uncertainty, the diagnosis appears quite clear.

With regard to her social functioning, Mrs Wright has shown a degree of indifference to markedly unsatisfactory living conditions over several years, and has lately tolerated having insufficient money to heat and light her home. Emily has been living with foster parents for the past one year. Her son, Graham, aged 19 years, lives with her. Her description of her daily activities is unremarkable, but I suspect that it is erroneous.

There is a great deal of background information that we need to gather, and Carol Penley is going to do this over the next few weeks. The really important thing is to engage with this lady. We are going to try and help her sort out her benefits, and get an emergency payment before the Christmas break. I don't think that her primary problem has anything to do with alcohol. She is showing unequivocal symptoms of chronic schizophrenia, with a longer-term history that is compatible with that diagnosis. I don't think that there is any great urgency in getting her to take medication. Once we have sorted out some practical problems and formed a relationship with her, it will be easier to work on improving her mental state. I will review her early in the New Year, and I will let you know what happens next.

Yours sincerely,

At the time of writing, audio-typing is the predominant method of producing letters. Dictaphones are small bits of equipment that seem to have a dispropor-tionate capacity to intimidate doctors. Consequently, doctors talk into them very quietly and quickly, which is exactly the opposite of what secretaries like. Slow clear speech makes an enormous difference. As far as possible, one should dictate the punctuation, as this makes it clearer to the secretary what you mean. You should break up the letter with paragraphs, as these make letters easier to read. Words that are unusual should be spelt out, including unusual names. When you're not speaking, stop the tape running, as long gaps are awkward on play back. When the letter is finished, say so, and when you've finished dictating, state that the tape is finished (failing to do so regularly risks the secretary missing a letter and wiping the tape). When the letter comes back for signing, always check it and correct errors. Especially look out for errors in drug doses, and bear in mind that even the most efficient secretary occasionally misses a 'not' and inadvertently reverses the meaning of a whole letter.

No one can automatically write good letters. This comes with practice. Following these points will however help considerably, and will make the team-secretary's life easier. It is worth nurturing the secretary. No other single individual can have such an impact in making your working life more pleasant or, if provoked, a lot more difficult.

Reports

Report writing is an intrinsic part of most psychiatrists' work. Many of these are quite straightforward, for example, reports to insurance companies. Others, especially court reports, are much more complex.

The first thing to think about in writing a report is whether you have permission from the patient or not. Not all reports require the patient's consent. For example, reports to mental health tribunals considering appeals against detention do not require patient consent. Most types of reports do require such permission, however, which should normally be obtained in writing.

The next question is 'What does the agency requesting this report need to know, and how much specialist knowledge are they likely to have?' Generally speaking, one should only reveal the minimum amount of confidential information necessary, even where you have permission from the patient. This is not to say that one should ever conceal relevant information, no matter how unpalatable. However, permission is often given under a degree of duress (for example, you only get your benefits if you reveal your psychiatric history), and it is wrong to needlessly expose that which is confidential.

In writing reports, psychiatric terminology has to be explained or turned into more ordinary language. There is no point in reporting something that the third party is unable to understand.

Major reports, usually to courts or mental health tribunals, should follow a set of well-established principles:

- No matter who has requested a report, your duty is to give as dispassionate an account and opinion as possible. In court reports, your duty is to the court. You should never get involved in a rhetorical process, nor alter your opinions to the convenience of one side or the other. If you are unable to form an opinion, or if you are unable to choose between two different ways of interpreting the situation, you should say so.
- It is conventional to refer to the subject by their full name throughout court reports. It is not necessary to follow this convention in other reports.

- The report should start with a statement as to who has requested the report, and the purpose of it. If you have been asked to comment on certain aspects of the situation, this should be stated at the outset.
- In some reports (especially where you are acting as an expert witness), it is necessary to set out your qualifications and experience. You need to be clear with whoever has requested the report whether you need to include a short resumé.
- Next, there should be a description of the evidence that you have drawn upon in preparing the report. This might be your experience of treating the patient over a specific length of time, or a single interview specifically for the purpose of preparing the report. In the latter case, you should make clear to the patient at the outset why you are seeing them and that anything they say may appear in the report. The fact that the patient was so warned should be stated in the report.
- Any records, reports, witness statements, documents or relevant interviews with third parties that have contributed towards the formation of your opinion should be listed.
- In the body of the report, it is extremely important to separate facts from opinions. The main part of the report should start with a factual account of the index events (admission to hospital or a criminal offence, for example), usually followed by the patient's account. In court reports, the offence should be referred to as 'the present alleged offence' even where the person intends to plead guilty.
- There should usually then be a psychiatric history followed by the background history. This need not necessarily be set out as fully as it would be in a clinical letter. There, however, needs to be sufficient information to allow the reader to understand exactly why you have reached the conclusions you have. This section should not include opinions, though you can report historically what your opinion was at a particular time. For example, you can state that you admitted the patient because at that time it was your opinion that they were depressed.
- There should be a description of the patient's mental state during the interview, usually the most recent interview that has occurred. Technical terms, such as 'delusions of reference' should be explained in parentheses '(the false belief that neutral material has a specific personal message)' or should be followed by a clear example from the patient's mental state examination.
- If there are complex issues or major ambiguities, it can be helpful to have a section marked 'Discussion', setting out the variety of ways in which the situation can be interpreted, allowing clarification before you express an opinion.

- Conclusions should be so headed, listed and numbered (this makes discussion of the report much easier in formal proceedings). Each numbered paragraph should contain one aspect of one's opinion, with the prelude 'In my opinion ...'. The listed opinions should move from the general to the particular, for example from whether the patient is under disability with respect to his trial, whether they have a mental illness, whether there are further psychiatric disorders present, whether there are physical factors of note, any circumstantial factors of relevance and the relationship between the mental disorder(s) and the person's behaviour, ending with any recommendations.
- You should not express an opinion outside of your professional expertise, no matter how obvious. If an opinion is based upon your general medical knowledge rather than specific psychiatric knowledge, you should say so.
- Court reports should end with a statement that the contents are true to the best of your knowledge and belief, and that you are content for the report to be placed before the court.

The real test of a psychiatric court report is whether you get asked to attend court or not. A well-written report about less serious offences will normally avoid you having to appear, as the report will be easy to understand and there will be little that the lawyers will feel able to challenge.

Reports often attract a fee for preparation, but one is mostly, in any case, more or less obliged to write them. It is easiest if one learns how to write them early in one's career, which normally means asking supervising consultants if you can write tribunal reports. It is true that the task is burdensome to begin with, but this is the only way of acquiring the necessary skills.

But the patient might read it ...

These days, patients are liable to read just about anything that a psychiatrist writes about them. This only matters if you are in the habit of being disparaging about patients in letters or if you do not discuss your conclusions or your plans with them. There are a tiny handful of situations where the latter might be justified, and none at all where the former is appropriate. With the introduction of the right to see clinic letters, there was a good deal of talk amongst psychiatrists about keeping 'double records' or changing the content of letters in some other way. In fact, most patients are not overly concerned to see letters. When they are, it often indicates that something has gone wrong with the relationship with the writer or the intended recipient. However, there is nothing wrong with people wanting to see letters and notes. In fact, it is a little surprising that doctors ever thought that it was acceptable to routinely write about people without their knowledge and in the absence of any right to know what had been written. If there are statements or conclusions in reports or letters that you are uncomfortable about the patient seeing, then it can be important to understand why this is so. In general, it is better for you to tell patients face-to-face what you have written, no matter how uncomfortable this might be. Truthfulness, openness and frankness are well recognised to be important in relationships in general, and are no less important in clinical relationships.

Main points in this chapter

1. Note-keeping, letters and reports are important. They are tedious tasks, but the skills can only be developed with thought and practice.
2. An awareness of the purpose of these documents is helpful.
3. Clarity of writing is improved if you bear in mind the recipient's needs, including any limitations to their knowledge of psychiatry.
4. Generally speaking, it is helpful to clearly separate fact from observation and opinion.
5. If you cannot share everything in a document with the patient, there is either something wrong in your relationship with the patient or they represent a high risk of an unusual type.

Afterword: getting alongside patients

Working in mental health is not a good way to get rich. Efforts to make a lot of money through psychiatry tend to take practitioners into ethically dubious territory. In every other respect, however, a career in mental health can be incredibly rewarding. Working as a psychiatrist can offer an extraordinarily rich experience and an unrivalled window into some of the most hidden aspects of human existence. The work can be intellectually demanding, stressful and frustrating, but it is never, ever, boring.

Two things become increasingly evident as you become more experienced. Firstly, it becomes obvious that the way that you deal with patients is at least as important as what you do by way of technical intervention. The second is that over time you encounter many people who overcome devastating mental illnesses with their dignity and self-respect intact; people who may still need the assistance of professionals from time to time, but who have learned to manage their mental illness, and in doing so, have recovered. To be of assistance in this process is a humbling experience.

Psychiatry: far from perfect ...

One of the things that makes psychiatry so interesting is that it is full of ambiguities. Working as a psychiatrist routinely presents you with dilemmas that defy simple or formulaic resolution. Dealing with such situations demands creativity and, in the absence of a right answer, you are bound to get things wrong sometimes. Working in psychiatry teaches you that the human spirit is an awesome thing, which can survive the severest mental illness. Unfortunately you also learn that it can be crushed by other people, even when they are well-intentioned. It takes courage to acknowledge that your own mistakes some times have this effect.

Organised psychiatry has been involved in some highly questionable activities in its short history (though in all likelihood individual doctors thought they were doing the right thing at the time). Psychiatrists were deeply involved in the eugenic projects of the first half of the twentieth century. They presided over forced sterilization programmes in the USA in the mistaken belief that they would thus eliminate mental illness from the population (Kelves, 1986). They participated in selecting people for death in the Nazi camps, sometimes in the belief that they were saving other lives (Lifton, 1988). In the 1950s and 1960s, they exposed patients to treatments, such as insulin therapy and narcosis, which they knew were dangerous. Unfortunately they also turned out to be ineffective. In the Soviet Union, as recently as the 1980s, psychiatry was misused for political purposes through construing dissent as psychopathology.

Psychiatry is not alone in having such a history. Social work, psychology and psychoanalysis all have corresponding histories that, in retrospect, are shameful and indefensible. Social values are unstable, and no doubt some aspects of modern practice will appear wrong in the near future. It is difficult for anyone to protect themselves against the risk of the retrospective condemnation of history. We should, nonetheless, try to avoid causing harm in the here and now.

Whilst the examples of the psychiatric abuse cited may seem extreme, distant and unrelated to modern psychiatric practice, psychiatry is not yet in the clear. Our capacity to do harm has not been eliminated. At the time of writing, organised psychiatry in the UK is taking a principled stand against governmental attacks on the civil liberties of the mentally disordered. The outcome is highly uncertain, and it is quite likely that, in the near future, individual psychiatrists will confront a conflict between their ethical and their legal duties.

Psychiatry can have more pervasive adverse effects. We stand accused of collusion with the medicalisation of everyday life. For example, the development of the concept of post-traumatic stress disorder (PTSD) has been criticised as an unhelpful extension of the disease metaphor (Summerfield, 2001). We tend to agree with this critique, and, in our opinion, the problems are not hypothetical.

If distress in the face of adverse social conditions is construed as an illness, with a technical solution that can only be delivered by experts, then there is an inevitable penalty for the sufferer in terms of personal helplessness. This encourages a victim mentality, in which people are angry at having been wronged, but look outside of themselves and their community for reparation and 'cure'. This is not to minimise the suffering of, for example, those who have been traumatised in war zones or by awful events in their lives. Nor are we dismissive of efforts to help people who cannot, in the fullness of time, recover emotionally. However, our hearts sink every time we hear on the news that teams of counsellors have been sent in to the aftermath of a catastrophe. Not only is there evidence that psychotherapeutic intervention can be harmful under these circumstances (Kenardy, 2000), but there is also a powerful message to society at large that recovery depends on the help of professionals, discouraging personal autonomy in the face of adversity.

The legitimate role of mental health services is to help people overcome mental illness. Sadly, if Karl Marx were still alive, he might well conclude that medication and counselling, rather than religion, is now the opium of the people, stifling their drive to improve their situation for themselves. Like the purveyors of opium, the pharmaceutical industry, the psychotherapeutic establishment and organised psychiatry might have some difficulty in persuading him that their efforts at easing the pains of living are altruistic rather than self-serving.

No one has all the answers as far as treating mental illness is concerned. If any one treatment were substantially better than any other, then there would not be such a range of treatments available. However, individual practitioners tend to become very attached to a particular approach. Unfortunately, there is a tendency to join a faction, and then to exaggerate the advantages of one's own approach and to minimise the strengths of other approaches. This creates the caricature of the 'biological psychiatrist' and the 'psychotherapeutic psychiatrist'. One of us gave up regarding himself as a psychotherapeutic psychiatrist after a trainee told him: 'The things you talk about are much more interesting than Dr X (*avowedly biological psychiatrist*), but the things you do are exactly the same'.

In a world where the ultimate causes of mental illness are obscure, and where all treatments have significant drawbacks, it is only ethical and fair to patients to be clear and open about this. To claim otherwise, to assert that particular drugs or psychotherapies hold the solution to some or all mental health problems, is to become a charlatan.

... but sometimes helpful, nonetheless

Fortunately, the divisions and disputes in the mental health community that have been so prominent in the past have lessened considerably in recent years. Indeed, there is reasonable consensus that psychiatrists are necessary (which is reassuring). Social psychiatry has gone out of fashion as a research area and as a research paradigm. This has occurred in the face of the relentless advance of the 'biological revolution' in the USA, and the expansion of the indications for CBT. Social psychiatry research tends to be large scale and expensive, and it generates few commercial opportunities. It is therefore difficult to get funding for it. However, social psychiatry is the dominant (though implicit) model for clinical psychiatrists, especially for those who work with deprived populations. There are a number of advantages to social psychiatry as a working model. It is pragmatic and eclectic. It does not demand adherence to any particular scientific religion. It is concerned with those factors that are realities in people's lives, rather than intangibles such as neurotransmitters or very rapid automatic thoughts outside of awareness. It can incorporate scientific advances without a paradigm shift, and it is as accessible to patients and families as it is to professionals, because you do not need a Ph.D. to understand it.

There is a growing consensus amongst professionals, patients, carers and even policy makers as to what type of psychiatrist is helpful. This is implicit in UK policy documents such as the National Institute for Clinical Excellence guidelines on the treatment of schizophrenia (NCCMH, 2002). When you talk to patients, they are generally clear about what they want in a psychiatrist, and their requirements are not unreasonable. Oddly, zealous attachment to a particular approach is not one of the things they want, though competence definitely is.

It is clear that patients like psychiatrists who are straight-talking, open, warm and engaging. They like doctors who can talk to them without being patronising or using jargon, but who, nonetheless, involve them in decision-making. People like to be treated as autonomous adults, with dignity and respect. Patients tend to like team working if it involves consistent individuals, and tend not to want to see the psychiatrist as often as the psychiatrist wants to see them. People like to learn to manage their own problems, and often recognise that dependency, though comfortable, is damaging.

A lot of doctors like hospitals, and some go misty eyed at the mention of the closed asylum in which they used to work. Very few patients have a similar attitude. In fact, what patients object to more than anything else is being treated in hospitals. Most patients would prefer to avoid admission if humanly possible, and are delighted when you make efforts to manage acute episodes of illness in their own home.

Above all, people are generally incredibly forgiving of their psychiatrists when they make mistakes or have made a difficult decision such as to detain them. There are two things that make a big difference under these circumstances: the first is if you can say that you are sorry, even if you also have to acknowledge that under the same circumstances you would do the same thing again; the second is if the patient can understand why you did what you did, and see that you did your best.

Good psychiatrists bring their humanity to their work. This allows the patient to relate to another real human being, the dyad thus sharing not just human failings, but also human strengths. There is a penalty for the doctor, because being emotionally engaged to people suffering from mental illness is distressing. However, it is also worthwhile, because it allows you to get alongside the patient, with a facilitative, not a dependent, relationship. It is this that allows the professional to assist, rather than impede, recovery.

References

Ackerman, P.T., Newton, J.E.O., McPherson, W.B. *et al.* (1998). Prevalence of post-traumatic stress disorder and other psychiatric diagnoses in three groups of abused children (sexual, physical and both). *Child Abuse and Neglect*, **22**, 759–74.

American Psychiatric Association (1994). *Diagnostic and Statistical Manual of Mental Disorders*, 4th edn. Washington: American Psychiatric Association.

Anthony, J.C., LeResche, L., Niaz, U. *et al.* (1982). Limits of the 'Mini-Mental State' as a screening test for dementia and delirium among hospital patients. *Psychological Medicine*, **12**, 397–408.

Bentall, R.P. (1992). A proposal to classify happiness as a psychiatric disorder. *Journal of Medical Ethics*, **18**, 94–8.

Brennan, P.A., Grekin, E.R. and Vanman, E.J. (2000). Major mental disorders and crime in the community. In *Violence among the Mentally Ill* (ed. P. Hodgins). Dordrecht: Kluwer Academic, pp. 3–18.

Clare, A.W. (1980). *Psychiatry in Dissent: Controversial Issues in Thought and Practice*, 2nd edn. London: Routledge.

Cleckley, H. (1988). *The Mask of Sanity*, 5th edn. Augusta, GA: Emily S Cleckley.

Cooper, J.E., Kendell, R.E., Gurland, B.J. *et al.* (1972). *Psychiatric Diagnosis in New York and London*. Maudsley Monograph No. 20. Oxford: Oxford University Press.

Cutting, J. (1990). *The Right Cerebral Hemisphere and Psychiatric Disorders*. Oxford: Oxford University Press.

Durkheim, E. (1951). *Suicide: A Study in Sociology* (ed. G. Simpson and J.A. Spaulding). New York: The Free Press.

Edwards, G. and Gross, M.M. (1976). Alcohol dependence: provisional description of a clinical syndrome. *British Medical Journal*, **1**, 1058–61.

Fink, M. and Taylor, M.A. (2003). *Catatonia: A Clinician's Guide to Diagnosis and Treatment*. Cambridge: Cambridge University Press.

Fish, F. (1985). *Clinical Psychopathology*, 2nd edn. Bristol: Wright.

Garety, P.A. (1985). Delusions: problems in definition and measurement. *British Journal of Clinical Psychology*, **58**, 25–34.

General Medical Council (2001). *Good Medical Practice*. London: GMC.

Hare, R.D. (1991). *The Hare Psychopathy Checklist – Revised*. Toronto: Multi-Health Systems.

Illich, I. (2001). *Limits to Medicine: Medical Nemesis*. New York: Marion Boyars.

Joukamaa, M., Heliovaara, M., Kneckt, P. *et al.* (2001). Mental disorders and cause-specific mortality. *British Journal of Psychiatry*, **179**, 498–502.

Kelves, D.J. (1986). *In the Name of Eugenics: Genetics and the Uses of Human Heredity*. London: Penguin.

Kenardy, J. (2000). The current status of psychological debriefing. *British Medical Journal*, **321**, 1032–3.

Kendell, R.E. (1976). The classification of depression: a review of contemporary confusion. *British Journal of Psychiatry*, **129**, 15–28.

Kendell, R.E., Brockington, I.F. and Leff, J.P. (1979). Prognostic implications of six alternative definitions of schizophrenia. *Archives of General Psychiatry*, **36**, 25–31.

Krawiecka, M., Goldberg, D. and Vaughan, M. (1977). A standardised psychiatric assessment scale for rating chronic psychotic patients. *Acta psychiatrica scandinavica*, **55**, 299–308.

Laing, R.D. (1990). *The Divided Self: An Existential Study in Sanity and Madness*. London: Penguin.

Lifton, R.J. (1988). *The Nazi Doctors: Medical Killing and the Psychology of Genocide*. New York: Basic Books.

Lishman, W.A. (1997). *Organic Psychiatry: The Psychological Consequences of Cerebral Disorder*. Oxford: Blackwell Science.

Mullen, P.E., Burgess, P., Wallace, C. *et al.* (2000). Community care and criminal offending in schizophrenia. *Lancet*, **355**, 1827–8.

National Collaborating Centre for Mental Health (2002). *Schizophrenia: Core Interventions in the Treatment and Management of Schizophrenia in Primary and Secondary Care*. London: NICE.

Ritchie, J., Dick, D. and Lingham, R. (1994). *Report of the Inquiry into the Care and Treatment of Christopher Clunis*. London: HMSO.

Romme, M. and Escher, S., eds. (1993). *Accepting Voices*. London: MIND Publications.

Schneider, K. (1959). *Clinical Psychopathology*. New York: Grune and Stratton.

Summerfield, D. (2001). The invention of post-traumatic stress disorder and the social usefulness of a psychiatric category. *British Medical Journal*, **322**, 95–8.

Taylor, P.J. and Gunn, J. (1999). Homicides by people with mental illness: myth and reality. *British Journal of Psychiatry*, **174**, 9–14.

van Os, J., Hanssen, M., Bijl, R.V. and Ravelli, A. (2000). Strauss (1969) revisited: a psychosis continuum in the general population? *Schizophrenia Research*, **45**, 11–20.

Webster, R. (1995). *Why Freud Was Wrong: Sin, Science and Psychoanalysis.* London: HarperCollins.

World Health Organization (1992). *Classification of Mental and Behavioural Disorders: Clinical Descriptions and Diagnostic Guidelines*, 10th edn. Geneva: WHO.

Zigmond, A.S. and Snaith, R.P. (1983). The hospital anxiety and depression scale. *Acta psychiatrica scandinavica*, **67**, 361–70.

Index